Menopause
for the MRCOG
and Beyond

Published titles in the MRCOG and Beyond series

Antenatal Disorders for the MRCOG and Beyond *by Andrew Thomson and Ian Greer*

Fetal Medicine for the MRCOG and Beyond *by Alan Cameron, Lena Macara, Janet Brennand and Peter Milton*

Gynaecological and Obstetric Pathology for the MRCOG *by Harold Fox and C. Hilary Buckley, with a chapter on Cervical Cytology by Dulcie V Coleman*

Gynaecological Oncology for the MRCOG and Beyond *edited by David Luesley and Nigel Acheson*

Gynaecological Urology for the MRCOG and Beyond *by Simon Jackson, Meghana Pandit and Alexandra Blackwell*

Haemorrhage and Thrombosis for the MRCOG and Beyond *edited by Anne Harper*

Intrapartum Care for the MRCOG and beyond *by Thomas F. Baskett and Sabaratnam Arulkumaran, with a chapter on Neonatal Resuscitation by John McIntyre and a chapter on Perinatal Loss by Carolyn Basak*

Management of Infertility for the MRCOG and Beyond, second edition, *edited by Siladitya Bhattacharya and Mark Hamilton*

Medical Genetics for the MRCOG and Beyond *by Michael Connor*

Menstrual Problems for the MRCOG *by Mary Ann Lumsden, Jane Norman and Hilary Critchley*

Neonatology for the MRCOG *by Peter Dear and Simon Newell*

Paediatric and Adolescent Gynaecology for the MRCOG and Beyond *by Anne S Garden and Joanne Topping*

Psychological Disorders in Obstetrics and Gynaecology for the MRCOG and Beyond *edited by Khaled M K Ismmail, Ilana Crome and P M Shaughn O'Brien*

Reproductive Endocrinology for the MRCOG and Beyond *edited by Adam Balen*

The MRCOG: A Guide to the Examination, third edition, *edited by William L Ledger and Michael G Murphy*

Forthcoming titles in the series

Early Pregnancy Issues

Molecular Medicine

Menopause for the MRCOG and Beyond

Second Edition

Margaret Rees MA DPhil FRCOG
Reader in Reproductive Medicine, Honorary Consultant in Medical
Gynaecology, John Radcliffe Hospital, Oxford and Visiting Professor,
Faculty of Medicine, University of Glasgow

Series Editor: Jenny Higham MD, FRCOG, FFFP, ILTM
Professor and Consultant Gynaecologist and
Head of Undergraduate Medicine, Faculty of Medicine,
Imperial College London

RCOG PRESS

Published by the **RCOG Press**
at the Royal College of Obstetricians and Gynaecologists
27 Sussex Place, Regent's Park, London NW1 4RG

www.rcog.org.uk

Registered charity no. 213280

First published 2002. This edition 2008

ISBN 978-1-904752-44-8

Cover illustration: Coloured scanning electron micrograph of the postmenopausal oviduct (fallopian tube) lining of a 63 year old woman. Seen here are ciliated cells, whose fine cilia (yellow) beat rhythmically to help propel ova from the ovaries to the uterus, and secretory cells (blue), which maintain a moist environment and provide nutrients for the ova. Magnification: x 2000 at 6 x 7 cm size. © 2008 Prof. P. Motta, Dept. Of Anatomy, University, 'La Sapienza', Rome, Science Photo Library.

RCOG Editor: Jane Moody
Design/typesetting: Tony Crowley
Index: Liza Furnival, Medical Indexing Ltd
Printed in the UK by Latimer Trend & Company Limited, Estover Road, Plymouth, Devon PL6 7PY.

Contents

Preface

The menopause remains a time of transition for women and brings many issues of interest to the gynaecologist. Although recent years have seen a substantial change in the attitude to prescribing hormone replacement therapy, there is a need for all those involved with women of the age group to be well informed. This is an authoritative guide, written by an author, Margaret Rees, who has a tremendous national and international reputation in the field. This volume covers the controversies in the field and, importantly, all aspects that a woman is likely to enquire about during a consultation. The gynaecologist is expected to be knowledgeable about the options, both medical and alternative – both are comprehensively reviewed here. The final chapter deals with women who have more complex problems and their management. All in all, a hugely useful read, both for examination preparation and to update the practitioner.

Jenny Higham
Series Editor

Abbreviations

aPL	antiphospholipid
BEPS	benign edematous polysynovitis syndrome
BMD	bone mineral density
CaD	calcium and vitamin D
CHD	coronary heart disease
CI	confidence interval
DCIS	ductal carcinoma *in situ*
DHEA	dehydroepiandrosterone
DMPA	depot medroxyprogesterone acetate
DXA	dual energy X-ray absorptiometry
EPT	estrogen and progestogen therapy
GnRH	gonadotrophin-releasing hormone
FSH	follicle-stimulating hormone
HDL-C	high-density lipoprotein C
HERS	Heart and Estrogen/progestin Replacement Study
HR	hazard ratio
HRT	hormone replacement therapy
IVF	*in vitro* fertilisation
LDL-C	low-density lipoprotein C
LH	luteinising hormone
MWS	Million Women Study
NHANES	National Health and Nutrition Examination Survey
NHSBSP	National Health Service Breast Screening Programme
OR	odds ratio
PEPI	Progestin Estrogen–Progestin Intervention
RANKL	receptor activator of nuclear factor kappa B ligand
RCT	randomised clinical trial
RR	relative risk
SD	standard deviation
SERM	selective estrogen-receptor modulator
SHBG	steroid hormone-binding globulin
SLE	systemic lupus erythematosus
TSH	thyroid-stimulating hormone
VTE	venous thromboembolism
WHI	Women's Health Initiative

1   Definitions and controversies

Introduction

The management of the menopausal and postmenopausal woman is an area where gynaecologists also become physicians, dealing not only with the consequences of ovarian failure but also of ageing. Estrogen deficiency affects many organ systems and a holistic approach is required. Postmenopausal health is a growing area of medicine as populations are ageing. The average age of the menopause, or last menstrual period, is 52 years. Current smoking, lower educational attainment, being separated/widowed/divorced, unemployment, Down syndrome and a history of heart disease are associated with earlier natural menopause, while parity, prior use of oral contraceptives and Japanese race/ethnicity are associated with later age at natural menopause.

Definitions

Various definitions are in use and are detailed in Box 1.

Stages of reproductive ageing

A staging system that uses the final or last menstrual period as the key event to describe reproductive ageing was proposed by the Stages of Reproductive Aging Workshop. In this system, five stages precede and two stages follow the final menstrual period. Stages −5 to −3 encompass the reproductive interval, stages −2 and −1 are the menopausal transition and stages 1 and 2 are the postmenopause. After menarche (stage −5), it usually takes several years for regular menstrual cycles to become established. Menstrual periods should then occur every 21–35 days for a number of years (stages −4 and −3). A woman's menstrual cycles remain regular in stage −2 (early menopausal transition) but the duration changes by 7 days or more (cycles are now every 24 days instead of every 31 days). Stage −1 (late menopausal transition) is characterised by two or more missed periods and at least one intermenstrual interval of 60 days or more. Stage +1 (early) and +2 (late) encompass the postmenopause. The early postmenopause is defined as 5 years since the final menstrual period and the late postmenopause thereafter until death.

BOX 1. DEFINITIONS OF MENOPAUSE

Menopause
The permanent cessation of menstruation that results from loss of ovarian follicular activity. Natural menopause is recognised after 12 consecutive months of amenorrhoea for which no other obvious pathological or physiological cause is present. Thus, the menopause is only known with certainty 1 year after the event. No adequate biological marker exists.

Perimenopause
Includes the period beginning with the first clinical, biological and endocrinological features of the approaching menopause, such as vasomotor symptoms and menstrual irregularity and ends 12 months after the last menstrual period.

Premenopause
A term often used ambiguously to refer to the 1–2 years immediately before the menopause or to the whole of the reproductive period before the menopause. Currently, this term is recommended to be used in the latter sense, encompassing the entire reproductive period from menarche to the final menstrual period.

Postmenopause
Should be defined from the final menstrual period regardless of whether the menopause was induced or spontaneous.

Menopausal transition
The period of time before the final menstrual period when variability in the menstrual cycle usually is increased.

Climacteric
The phase marking the transition from the reproductive state to the non-reproductive state.

Climacteric syndrome
The climacteric is sometimes but not always associated with symptoms such as hot flushes. When this occurs, the term 'climacteric syndrome' may be used.

Induced menopause
The cessation of menstruation that follows bilateral oophorectomy or iatrogenic ablation of ovarian function by chemotherapy, radiotherapy or treatment with gonadotrophin-releasing hormone analogues. In the absence of surgery, induced menopause may be permanent or temporary.

The ageing population: postmenopausal health as a public health issue

A woman's average life expectancy at birth in the UK is currently 81 years; it is increasing and is estimated to reach 85 years by 2031. Women live longer than men. Worldwide, increasing life expectancy and decreasing fertility rates mean that the number of people older than 65 years is projected to grow considerably in absolute and relative terms. In 2002, 440 million people were older than 65 years; this was about 7% of the total population. This figure is projected to increase rapidly and it is estimated that the elderly will comprise nearly 17% of the world's population in 2050. The percentage of elderly people is higher in the countries that make up the developed world and very low in Africa and the Near East; thus, maintaining the health of postmenopausal women is an extremely important public health issue.

Controversies

Management of the menopause and postmenopausal health has become extremely controversial following publication of the US Women's Health Initiative (WHI) studies and the UK Million Women Study (MWS). Both these studies were undertaken in women aged over 50 years of age.

WOMEN'S HEALTH INITIATIVE STUDIES

The WHI studies were designed to examine strategies for the prevention and control of some of the most common causes of morbidity and mortality among postmenopausal women aged 50–79 years, including cancer, cardiovascular disease and osteoporotic fractures. It involved a randomised clinical trial (RCT) in 68 132 women and an observational study. Women were identified from the general population living in proximity to any of the 40 participating clinical centres throughout the USA. The observational study included 93 676 women recruited from the same population base as the RCT.

The RCT evaluated the health benefits and risks of four distinct interventions:
- dietary modification
- two types of hormone replacement therapy (HRT) in a randomised placebo-controlled trial
- calcium/vitamin D supplementation.

The HRT regimens were conjugated equine estrogens 0.625 mg in 10 739 (39.3%) women who had undergone hysterectomy and conjugated equine estrogens 0.625 mg combined with continuous medroxyprogesterone acetate 2.5 mg in 16 608 (60.7%) women who had not had a hysterectomy. The same dose was used for all age groups.

Enrolment into WHI began in 1993 and concluded in 1998. Intervention activities in the estrogen plus progestogen HRT component of the trial ended early on 8 July 2002, when evidence had accumulated that the risks exceeded the benefits in the group overall. Intervention activities in the estrogen-alone component of the trial also ended early, on 29 February 2004. The other two studies ended on 31 March 2005. Nonintervention follow-up on participating women is planned until 2010, giving an average follow-up duration of about 13 years in the RCT and 12 years in the observational study.

The RCT used a 'partial factorial' design. Participating women were randomised to either the dietary modification or HRT interventions, or both dietary modification and HRT. The dietary modification component randomly assigned 48835 eligible women to either a sustained low-fat eating pattern (40%) or self-selected dietary behaviour (60%), with breast cancer and colorectal cancer as designated primary outcomes and coronary heart disease (CHD) as a secondary outcome. The nutritional goals for women assigned to the dietary modification intervention group were to reduce total dietary fat to 20% and saturated fat to 7% of corresponding daily calories and, secondarily, to increase daily servings of vegetables and fruits to at least five and of grain products to at least six, and to maintain these changes throughout the trial intervention period. The HRT studies had CHD as the primary outcome, with hip and other fractures as secondary outcomes and with breast cancer as a primary adverse outcome. A total of 8050 women were randomised to both the dietary modification and HRT trials.

At their 1-year anniversary from dietary modification and/or HRT trial enrolment, all women in the RCT were further screened for possible randomisation in the calcium and vitamin D (CaD) component, a randomised, double-blind, placebo-controlled trial of 1000 mg elemental calcium plus 400 international units of vitamin D3 daily, versus placebo. Hip fracture was the designated primary outcome for the CaD component, with other fractures and colorectal cancer as secondary outcomes. A total of 36282 (53.3% of RCT enrollees) were randomised to the CaD component.

Postmenopausal women who were screened for the RCT but proved to be ineligible or unwilling to be randomised were offered the opportunity to enrol in the observational study. The observational study was intended to provide additional knowledge about risk factors for a range of diseases, including cancer, cardiovascular disease and fractures. It has an emphasis on biological markers of disease risk and on risk factor changes as modifiers of risk.

The WHI studies also collected and stored biological materials. This included plasma and serum, as well as white blood cells for DNA extraction. It is hoped that these well-characterised specimens from the RCT and observational study cohorts will provide an extremely valuable resource for elucidating mechanisms that determine chronic disease risk, and for explaining RCT intervention effects.

Since initial publication of the results in the overall group, there have been many subsequent papers with subgroup analyses which have shown marked differences relevant to clinical practice (see Chapter 2).

The WHI trial has important limitations and a selection of comments is given below:

- The women were mainly from relatively older age groups: approximately 70% were over 65 years of age.
- The women were not generally healthy: approximately 8% had pre-existing coronary heart disease.
- Women without menopausal symptoms were in general recruited: only 10% had vasomotor symptoms.
- The women in the WHI trial thus did not represent the younger (under 60 years of age) healthy, postmenopausal women with vasomotor symptoms who are most commonly prescribed HRT and who are probably at much lower risk than suggested by the WHI trial.

MILLION WOMEN STUDY

The MWS is an observational study that evaluated the risk of cancer (such as breast, endometrial and ovarian) with respect to differences in HRT regimen and routes of administration (with the exception of vaginal preparations) in women aged 50–64 years. Women invited to attend the NHS Breast Screening Programme (NHSBSP) were sent a self-administered questionnaire that asked them to document details about personal medical history and lifestyle factors, including the use of HRT. The study data were recorded from these questionnaires (which were returned before initial mammography) and women were followed to determine the incidence of cancer and death. A total of 1 084 110 women were recruited between 1996 and 2001; around 50% had ever used HRT. The average duration of follow-up was 2.6 years. Several publications have questioned its design, analysis and conclusions and a selection of comments is given below:

- The representation of the sample is uncertain. Differences between women who did or did not attend for mammography or who agreed or declined to participate in the study cannot easily be controlled for.
- Use or non-use of HRT was established only at study entry and changes were not recorded during follow-up. Thus, there is uncertainty as to whether women switched preparations or started or stopped HRT during the study's follow-up period.

- Accuracy of recall of HRT use has been questioned. Validation of the questionnaire data was based on information obtained from only 570 women. Curiously, although the risk of endometrial cancer with unopposed estrogen is well established, 14 024 women who had not undergone hysterectomy were documented as having taken HRT that contained estrogen alone.
- Many differences were present when women who used and did not use HRT were compared and this required multiple adjustments.
- Mortality from breast cancer was assessed after an average of 4.1 years of follow up and on the basis of a total of 517 deaths; however, breast cancer was diagnosed very rapidly, after a mean of 1.2 years, and deaths occurred swiftly (within an average of 1.7 years). This can be attributed to an underestimation of the total duration of HRT use.
- The higher estimates of risk reported compared with those from the randomised WHI study – especially the estrogen-alone arm, which found a reduced risk – probably reflects the observational nature of the MWS and suggests that the latter study probably grossly overestimated the risk of breast cancer.

Further reading

Beral V, Bull D, Reeves G; Million Women Study Collaborators. Endometrial cancer and hormone-replacement therapy in the Million Women Study. *Lancet* 2005;365:1543–51.

Beral V; Million Women Study Collaborators, Bull D, Green J, Reeves G. Ovarian cancer and hormone replacement therapy in the Million Women Study. *Lancet* 2007;369:1703–10.

Davey DA. Hormone replacement therapy: time to move on? *J Br Menopause Soc* 2006;12:75–80.

Garton M. Breast cancer and hormone-replacement therapy: the Million Women Study. *Lancet* 2003;362:1328–31.

Gold EB, Bromberger J, Crawford S, Samuels S, Greendale GA, Harlow SD, et al. Factors associated with age at natural menopause in a multiethnic sample of midlife women. *Am J Epidemiol* 2001;153:865–74.

Government Actuary's Department [www.gad.gov.uk].

Hardy R, Kuh D. Social and environmental conditions across the life course and age at menopause in a British birth cohort study. *BJOG* 2005;112:346–54.

Harlow SD, Crawford S, Dennerstein L, Burger HG, Mitchell ES, Sowers MF; ReSTAGE Collaboration. Recommendations from a multi-study evaluation of proposed criteria for staging reproductive aging. *Climacteric* 2007;10:112–19.

Million Women Study Collaborators. Breast cancer and hormone-replacement therapy in the Million Women Study. *Lancet* 2003;362:419–27.

Prentice RL, Pettinger M, Anderson GL. Statistical issues arising in the Women's Health Initiative. *Biometrics* 2005;61:899–911.

Seltzer GB, Schupf N, Wu HS. A prospective study of menopause in women with Down syndrome. *J Intellect Disabil Res* 2001;45(Pt 1):1–7.

Speroff L. Clinical appraisal of the Women's Health Initiative. *J Obstet Gynaecol Res* 2005;31:80–93.

US Census Bureau. World Population Information [www.census.gov/ipc/www/world.html] accessed 24 May 2007.

Wanless D. Securing good care for older people. Taking a long term view. Wanless social care review [www.kingsfund.org.uk/resources/publications/securing_good.html].

Whitehead M, Farmer R. The Million Women Study: a critique. *Endocrine* 2004;24:187–93.

Women's Health Initiative Steering Committee. Effects of conjugated equine estrogen in postmenopausal women with hysterectomy: the Women's Health Initiative randomized controlled trial. *JAMA* 2004;291:1701–2.

Writing Group for the Women's Health Initiative Investigators. Risks and benefits of estrogen plus progestin in healthy postmenopausal women: principal results From the Women's Health Initiative randomized controlled trial. *JAMA* 2002;288:321–33.

2   Explaining risk

Women may be concerned about the risks of any particular treatment and, in the case of menopausal women, HRT in particular. This has not been helped by media scares. This chapter focuses on how to explain risk and the risks in certain clinical situations.

Relative risk, absolute risk, attributable risk

The terms 'relative risk', 'absolute risk' and 'attributable risk' can be confusing. An understanding of the precise definitions is important to judge the actual magnitude of risks involved.

Relative risk (RR) is the risk of an event (or of developing a disease) relative to exposure. Relative risk is a ratio of the probability of the event occurring in the exposed group versus the control (non-exposed) group. It is often used to present clinical trial data, where it is used to compare the risk of developing a disease in people receiving a treatment compared with those not receiving treatment (or receiving a placebo). However, it does not take into account the actual frequency of the condition in the untreated group. For example, a relative risk of 2 could describe something that increased the risk of a disease from one in a million to two in a million or something that increased the risk of a disease from four people in ten to eight people in ten. Thus 'absolute risk' and 'attributable risk', which take into account the frequency of the condition, are better methods of presenting the data.

Absolute risk is determined by multiplying the usual rate of the condition in the untreated group by the relative risk.

Attributable risk is an absolute measure of the excess risk attributed to treatment. It is calculated as the difference in risk of a particular condition between those who are treated and those who are not.

Odds and hazard ratios

Risk also can be expressed as odds and hazard ratios. The odds ratio (OR) is the odds of an event happening in the treated group expressed as a proportion of the odds of an event happening in the untreated group. When events are rare, the odds ratio is analogous to the relative risk but, as event rates increase, the odds ratio and relative risk diverge.

Hazard ratios (HR) are broadly equivalent to relative risk and are useful when the risk is not constant with respect to time. They use information collected at different times and were used in the publications from the WHI studies. The term typically is used in the context of survival over time. If the hazard ratio is 0.5, the relative risk of dying in one group is half the risk of dying in the other group.

Differences between regimens

Women may believe that the risks of HRT are the same for all regimens. This is not the case. There are differences between estrogen-alone HRT used in women who have had a hysterectomy versus combined HRT used in women with an intact uterus. There are also differences between oral and transdermal administration. Examples are given below.

ESTROGEN ALONE VERSUS COMBINED ESTROGEN–PROGESTOGEN COMBINED HRT

The examples given here come from the WHI randomised study.

Breast cancer

The risk of breast cancer in the estrogen-alone arm of the WHI study was lower than in the placebo group, which, in absolute numbers, represents four fewer cases at 50–59 years of age, five fewer at 60–69 years and one at 70–79 years per 1000 women on an intention to treat for 5 years. However, with combined therapy there was an excess risk, being three more cases at 50–59 years, four more at 60–69 years and seven more cases at 70–79 years (Table 1).

Table 1	Breast cancer risk per 1000 women from intention-to-treat analysis of 5 years of data from the Women's Health Initiative studies (adapted from Chlebowski *et al.*, 2003)			
Age range (years)	Risk of breast cancer/1000 women			
	Estrogen only		Continuous combined HRT	
	HR (95% CI)	Difference	HR (95% CI)	Difference
50–59	0.72 (0.43 to 1.21)	–4 (–7 to +3)	1.20 (0.80 to 1.82)	+3 (–3 to +11)
60–69	0.72 (0.49 to 1.07)	–5 (–9 to +1)	1.22 (0.90 to 1.66)	+4 (–2 to +12)
70–79	0.94 (0.56 to 1.60)	–1 (–9 to +12)	1.34 (0.88 to 2.04)	+7 (–2 to +21)
All	0.77 (0.59 to 1.01)	–4 (–7 to 0)	1.24 (1.01 to 1.54)	+4 (0 to +9)

Coronary heart disease

The combined WHI arm showed an early, albeit transient, increase in coronary events. Overall, there was no significant effect of HRT. The excess absolute risk at 50–59 years was 5, 60–69 years 1 and 70–79 years 23 cases of nonfatal myocardial infarction and death due to CHD/10 000 women/year. In the estrogen-alone study, a nonsignificant reduction in CHD was found, which was most marked in the younger (50–59 years) age group. In this subgroup, there was a significant reduction in a composite of coronary events and procedures and there were no significant increases in events in the older age groups. The reduced absolute risk at 50–59 years was 10 and at 60–69 years it was 5, with an excess risk of four cases in those aged 70–79 years.

Endometrial cancer

Unopposed estrogen replacement therapy increases endometrial cancer risk. Thus, progestogen is added in regimens for women with an intact uterus to reduce the risk. Most studies have shown that this excess risk with estrogen alone is not completely eliminated with monthly sequential progestogen addition, especially when continued for more than 5 years. This has also been found with long-cycle HRT. However, no increased risk of endometrial cancer has been found with continuous combined regimens and this is why these regimens are recommended for postmenopausal women.

ORAL VERSUS TRANSDERMAL THERAPY

Oral therapy is usually a first-line option because of cost. However, transdermal administration avoids the gut and first-pass effects on the liver. Thus, after oral administration, the dominant circulating estrogen is estrone, while after parenteral administration it is estradiol.

Substances normally synthesised in the liver, such as coagulation factors, may be affected differentially by oral or transdermal delivery. This is clinically relevant in women at risk of venous thromboembolism (VTE). A multicentre case–control study found that oral but not transdermal estrogen is associated with an increased VTE risk. Furthermore, transdermal estrogen does not appear to confer additional risk on women who carry a prothrombotic mutation.

Timing of treatment

CORONARY HEART DISEASE

The WHI studies included women who started HRT at various times after the menopause. Some started it within 10 years while others began after more than 20 years. Women in the WHI who started combined HRT

Table 2 Estimated absolute excess risk of CHD for women/10 000 person-years (data from Rossouw et al., 2007)

Years since menopause	Estimated absolute excess risk for CHD/10 000 person-years
< 10	–6
10–19	4
≥ 20	17

Table 3 Absolute excess risk of CHD/10 000 person-years in older age groups (data from Rossouw et al., 2007)

Age group (years)	Absolute excess risk for CHD/10 000 person-years	Hazard ratio (95% CI)
50–59	–2	0.93 (0.65–1.33)
60–69	–1	0.98 (0.79–1.21)
70–79	+19	1.26 (1.00–1.59)

within 10 years of the menopause had a lower risk of CHD than women who started later (Table 2). Combining the two HRT arms found that women who initiated hormone therapy closer to menopause tended to have reduced CHD risk compared with the increase in CHD risk among women more distant from menopause (Table 3) Furthermore, in the Nurses' Health Study, women beginning HRT near menopause had a significantly reduced risk of CHD (RR 0.66, 95% CI 0.54–0.80 for estrogen alone; RR0.72, 95% CI 0.56–0.92 for estrogen with progestogen).

DEMENTIA

While estrogen may delay or reduce the risk of Alzheimer's disease, it does not seem to improve established disease. It is unclear whether there is a critical age or duration of treatment for exposure to estrogen to have an effect in prevention but there may be a window of opportunity in the early postmenopause when the pathological processes that lead to Alzheimer's disease are being initiated and when HRT may have a preventive effect. WHI found a two-fold increased risk of dementia in women with both estrogen and progestogen and estrogen alone. However, this increased risk was only significant in the group of women over the age of 75 years.

Table 4	Age-specific probabilities of developing breast cancer (source: American Cancer Society. Breast Cancer Facts and Figures 2005–2006)	

Current age (years)	Probability of developing breast cancer in next 10 years
20	1/1985
30	1/229
40	1/68
50	1/37
60	1/26
70	1/24

PREMATURE MENOPAUSE

Women with premature ovarian failure are often confused about taking HRT, extrapolating findings from women in their 50s such as the WHI and MWS studies to apply to themselves. That they would normally be exposed to their own endogenous estrogen seems to be forgotten. A common fear is that of an increased risk of breast cancer. However, their risk of breast cancer is low and the available evidence shows that giving HRT below the age of 50 years does not increase breast cancer risk (Table 4). Regulatory bodies recommend the use of HRT in premature ovarian failure up till the average age of the natural menopause.

Balancing risks

Certain lifestyle factors increase risk of disease more than taking any medication such as HRT. The main example is breast cancer risk (see Chapter 9). Some factors, such as age, family history, early menarche, late menopause and being tall, are not modifiable. Others, such as obesity and alcohol consumption, are. Thus, consultations about postmenopausal health have to take a holistic approach and explore lifestyle and family history.

Further reading

American Cancer Society. Breast cancer facts and figures 2005–2006 [www.ca ncer.org/downloads/STT/CAFF2005BrFacspdf2005.pdf].

Anderson GL, Judd HL, Kaunitz AM, Barad DH, Beresford SA, Pettinger M, *et al;* Women's Health Initiative Investigators. Effects of estrogen plus progestin on gynecologic cancers and associated diagnostic procedures: the Women's Health Initiative randomized trial. *JAMA* 2003;290:1739–48.

Beral V, Bull D, Reeves G; Million Women Study Collaborators. Endometrial cancer and hormone-replacement therapy in the Million Women Study. *Lancet* 2005;365:1543–51.

Canonico M, Oger E, Plu-Bureau G, Conard J, Meyer G, Lévesque H, *et al;* Estrogen and Thromboembolism Risk (ESTHER) Study Group. Hormone therapy and venous thromboembolism among postmenopausal women: impact of the route of estrogen administration and progestogens: the ESTHER study. *Circulation* 2007;115:840–5.

Chlebowski RT, Hendrix SL, Langer RD, Stefanick ML, Gass M, Lane D, *et al;* WHI Investigators. Influence of estrogen plus progestin on breast cancer and mammography in healthy postmenopausal women: the Women's Health Initiative Randomized Trial. *JAMA* 2003;289:3243–53.

Espeland MA, Rapp SR, Shumaker SA, Brunner R, Manson JE, Sherwin BB, *et al;* Women's Health Initiative Memory Study. Conjugated equine estrogens and global cognitive function in postmenopausal women: Women's Health Initiative Memory Study. *JAMA* 2004;291:2959–68.

Ewertz M, Mellemkjaer L, Poulsen AH, Friis S, Sørensen HT, Pedersen L, *et al.* Hormone use for menopausal symptoms and risk of breast cancer. A Danish cohort study. *Br J Cancer* 2005;92:1293–7.

Grodstein F, Manson JE, Stampfer MJ. Hormone therapy and coronary heart disease: the role of time since menopause and age at hormone initiation. *J Women's Health* 2006;15:35–44.

Hsia J, Langer RD, Manson JE, Kuller L, Johnson KC, Hendrix SL, *et al.* Conjugated equine estrogens and coronary heart disease: the Women's Health Initiative. *Arch Intern Med* 2006;166:357–65.

Manson JE, Hsia J, Johnson KC, Rossouw JE, Assaf AR, Lasser NL, *et al;* Women's Health Initiative Investigators. Estrogen plus progestin and the risk of coronary heart disease. *N Engl J Med* 2003;349:523–34.

Prentice RL, Langer RD, Stefanick ML, Howard BV, Pettinger M, Anderson GL, *et al.* Combined analysis of Women's Health Initiative observational and clinical trial data on postmenopausal hormone treatment and cardiovascular disease. *Am J Epidemiol* 2006;163:589–99.

Rapp SR, Espeland MA, Shumaker SA, Henderson VW, Brunner RL, Manson JE, *et al.* Effect of estrogen plus progestin on global cognitive function in postmenopausal women: The Women's Health Initiative Memory Study: a randomized controlled trial. *JAMA* 2003;289:2663–72.

Rees M, Purdie DW. *Management of the Menopause. The Handbook.* 4th ed. London: RSM Press; 2006.

Rossouw JE, Prentice RL, Manson JE, Wu L, Barad D, Barnabei VM, *et al.* Postmenopausal hormone therapy and risk of cardiovascular disease by age and years since menopause. *JAMA* 2007;297:1465–77.

Shumaker SA, Legault C, Kuller L, Rapp SR, Thal L, Lane DS, *et al;* Women's Health Initiative Memory Study. Conjugated equine estrogens and incidence of probable dementia and mild cognitive impairment in postmenopausal women: Women's Health Initiative Memory Study. *JAMA* 2004;291:2947–58.

Shumaker SA, Legault C, Rapp SR, Thal L, Wallace RB, Ockene JK, *et al.* Estrogen plus progestin and the incidence of dementia and mild cognitive impairment in postmenopausal women: the Women's Health Initiative Memory Study: a randomized controlled trial. *JAMA* 2003;289:2651–62.

Stefanick ML, Anderson GL, Margolis KL, Hendrix SL, Rodabough RJ, Paskett ED, *et al.* Effects of conjugated equine estrogens on breast cancer and mammography screening in postmenopausal women with hysterectomy. *JAMA* 2006;295:1647–57.

Straczek C, Oger E, Yon de Jonage-Canonico MB, Plu-Bureau G, Conard J, Meyer G, *et al;* Estrogen and Thromboembolism Risk (ESTHER) Study Group. Prothrombotic mutations, hormone therapy, and venous thromboembolism among postmenopausal women: impact of the route of estrogen administration. *Circulation* 2005;112:3495–500.

Weiderpass E, Adami HO, Baron JA, Magnusson C, Bergström R, Lindgren A, *et al.* Risk of endometrial cancer following estrogen replacement with and without progestins. *J Natl Cancer Inst* 1999;91:1131–7.

Women's Health Initiative Steering Committee. Effects of conjugated equine estrogen in postmenopausal women with hysterectomy: the Women's Health Initiative randomized controlled trial. *JAMA* 2004;291:1701–12.

Writing Group for the Women's Health Initiative Investigators. Risks and benefits of estrogen plus progestin in healthy postmenopausal women: principal results From the Women's Health Initiative randomized controlled trial. *JAMA* 2002;288:321–33.

Zandi PP, Carlson MC, Plassman BL, Welsh-Bohmer KA, Mayer LS, Steffens DC, *et al;* Cache County Memory Study Investigators. Hormone replacement therapy and incidence of Alzheimer disease in older women: the Cache County Study. *JAMA* 2002;288:2123–9.

3 Systemic hormone replacement therapy

Many HRT preparations are available with different combinations, strengths and routes of administration. Various terms are used such as hormone therapy for estrogen therapy and EPT (estrogen and progestogen therapy) for combined preparations. Regimens may vary between countries.

HRT regimens

Hormone replacement therapy consists of estrogen alone in women who have had a hysterectomy but is combined with a progestogen in women with an intact uterus. Progestogens are given cyclically or continuously with the estrogen. Systemic estrogens can be delivered orally, transdermally (patch or gel) or subcutaneously (implant). Topical estrogens are given vaginally and these are discussed further in Chapter 4. Progestogens can be delivered orally, transdermally (patch) or directly into the uterus.

ESTROGENS

Two types of estrogen are available: synthetic and natural. Synthetic estrogens, such as ethinyl estradiol, are generally considered to be not suitable for HRT because of their greater metabolic impact except for women with premature ovarian failure (see Chapter 11). Natural estrogens include estradiol, estrone and estriol. These are synthesised from soya beans or yams and are chemically identical to the natural human hormones. Conjugated equine estrogens are derived from pregnant mares' urine. The active ingredients are primarily the sulphate esters of estrone, equilin sulphates, 17α-estradiol and 17β-estradiol.

Symptom control
Young women who experience a surgical menopause may initially need higher doses of estrogen to alleviate menopausal symptoms than their older counterparts; for example, 4 mg estradiol rather than 1 mg. Conversely, older women usually require lower doses to control their symptoms.

Table 5	Generally accepted minimum bone-sparing doses of estrogen
Estrogen preparation	*Dose*
Estradiol oral	1–2 mg
Conjugated equine estrogens	0.3–0.625 mg daily
Estradiol patch	25–50 micrograms
Estradiol gel	1–5 g*
Estradiol implant	50 mg every 6 months
* depending on preparation	

Osteoporosis

The generally accepted minimum bone-sparing doses of estrogen are listed in Table 5, although increasing evidence shows that even lower doses may be effective.

Progestogens

The progestogens used in HRT are also derived from plant sources, such as soy beans or yams. Currently, they are mainly given orally, although norethisterone and levonorgestrel are available in transdermal patches combined with estradiol and levonorgestrel can be delivered directly to the uterus. The intrauterine system delivers 20 micrograms/day of levonorgestrel to the endometrium and provides the progestogen component of HRT. This method of delivery also provides a solution to the problem of contraception in the perimenopause and is also the only way in which a 'no bleed' regimen can be achieved in perimenopausal women. A device that releases 10 micrograms/day has been evaluated for early postmenopausal women.

Progesterone, the native hormone, is formulated either as an oral tablet or a 4% vaginal gel but availability varies worldwide. A progesterone pessary for vaginal or rectal use is available but is currently not licensed for HRT. The classification of progestogens is shown in Box 2.

Tibolone

Tibolone is a synthetic steroid compound that itself is inert but is converted *in vivo* to metabolites with estrogenic, progestogenic and androgenic actions. It is classified as HRT in the British National Formulary. It is used in postmenopausal women who wish to have amenorrhoea and also used to treat vasomotor, psychological and libido problems. The daily dose is 2.5 mg. It conserves bone mass and reduces the risk of vertebral fracture.

BOX 2. CLASSIFICATION OF PROGESTOGENS

Progestogens structurally related to progesterone

1 Pregnane derivatives:

   a acetylated (also called 17α-hydroxyprogesterone derivatives): medroxyprogesterone acetate, megestrol acetate, cyproterone acetate)

   b non-acetylated: dydrogesterone

2 19-norpregnane derivatives (also called 19-norprogesterone derivatives):

   a acetylated: nomegestrol acetate

   b non-acetylated: trimegestone

Progestogens structurally related to testosterone (also called 19-nortestosterone derivatives)

1 Ethinylated:

   a estranes: norethisterone, ethynodiol diacetate

   b gonanes: levonorgestrel, norgestrel, desogestrel, gestodene, norgestimate

2 Non-ethinylated: dienogest, drospirenone

Androgens

Testosterone can be administered either as a patch or a subcutaneous implant. Androgens may be used to improve libido but are not successful in all women, as other factors, such as marital problems, may be involved. Testosterone gels currently are licensed for use in men.

ROUTES OF ADMINISTRATION

Oral administration is the usual chosen route because of cost and in most women there is no clear advantage in the non-oral routes. Non-oral routes avoid the gut and the first pass effects on the liver but all estrogens, regardless of the route of administration, eventually pass through the liver and are recycled by the enterohepatic circulation. After oral administration, the predominant circulating estrogen is estrone while after parenteral administration it is estradiol.

Transdermal systems

Two transdermal systems are available: patch and gel. Two patch technologies exist: alcohol-based reservoir patches, which have an adhesive outer ring, and matrix patches, in which the hormone is distributed evenly throughout the adhesive. Skin reactions are less common with matrix patches than with reservoir patches. Of the progestogens, currently only norethisterone and levonorgestrel are delivered transdermally in patches. At present, only estradiol is delivered in a gel.

Implants

Estradiol implants are crystalline pellets of estradiol that are inserted subcutaneously under local anaesthesia and release estradiol over many months. Implants have the advantage that, once inserted, the woman does not have to remember to take her drugs. A significant concern is tachyphylaxis, which may be defined as a recurrence of menopausal symptoms while the implant is still releasing adequate levels of estradiol. Another concern is that implants may remain effective for many years. A check on levels of estradiol in plasma before reimplantation should be considered, especially in women who return more frequently for treatment, to ensure that the pre-implantation level is in the normal premenopausal range (< 1000 pmol/l).

Adjusting regimens

ESTROGEN ALONE: WOMEN WHO HAVE HAD A HYSTERECTOMY

In general, women who have had a hysterectomy should be given estrogen alone and should have no need for a progestogen. There may be concerns about a remnant of endometrium in the cervical stump in women who have had a subtotal hysterectomy. If this is suspected, the presence or absence of bleeding induced by monthly sequential HRT may be a useful diagnostic test.

COMBINED ESTROGEN AND PROGESTOGEN: WOMEN WITH AN INTACT UTERUS

Progestogens are added to estrogens to reduce the increased risk of endometrial hyperplasia and carcinoma, which occurs with unopposed estrogen. Progestogen can be given 'sequentially' for 10–14 days every 4 weeks, for 14 days every 13 weeks or every day ('continuously'). The first regimen leads to monthly bleeds, the second to bleeds every 3 months and the last aims to achieve amenorrhoea and is also called 'no-bleed HRT'. Progestogen must be given to women who have undergone endometrial ablative techniques, as it cannot be assumed that all the endometrium has been removed.

MENOPAUSAL STATUS

Perimenopausal women

Sequential or cyclic therapy should be given to these women who have inherent ovarian activity. Alternatively intrauterine levonorgestrel can be given and this is especially useful in women with heavy menstrual bleeding or needing contraception. It is the only method of achieving 'no-bleed' HRT in the perimenopause. Continuous combined regimens should not be used in perimenopausal women because of the high risk of irregular bleeding. The options available are monthly cyclic or 3-monthly cyclic regimens. For women with infrequent menstruation and those who are intolerant of progestogens, a 3-monthly preparation can be considered. Only one such preparation is available in the UK at present: it contains estradiol valerate and medroxyprogesterone acetate.

Postmenopausal women

Women are considered to be postmenopausal 12 months after their last menstrual period. This definition is difficult to apply in clinical practice, especially in women who started HRT in the perimenopause or who are using intrauterine levonorgestrel. Pragmatically, menopausal status can be estimated from:

- age: it has been estimated that 80% of women will be postmenopausal by the age of 54 years
- previous amenorrhoea or increased levels of follicle-stimulating hormone (FSH): women who experienced 6 months of amenorrhoea or had increased levels of FSH in their mid-40s are likely to be postmenopausal after taking several years of monthly sequential HRT.

Continuous combined regimens should be used in postmenopausal women because of the lack of induced bleeding. Also, continuous combined treatment may have a reduced risk of endometrial cancer compared with sequential regimens. Continuous combined therapy induces endometrial atrophy. Intrauterine delivery of levonorgestrel can be continued but it may be technically more difficult to insert the intrauterine device as women become older.

Troubleshooting

STARTING HRT

Hot flushes, mood changes, tiredness, arthralgia and vaginal dryness may start several months or years before periods stop. There is no need to measure FSH levels to confirm ovarian failure in women over the age of 45 years presenting with such symptoms. Indeed, FSH values may be unhelpful because of marked fluctuations in the perimenopause. Amenorrhoea need not be awaited before HRT is started. The dose used should be tailored to control menopausal symptoms. When starting HRT, some women may experience breast tenderness, especially if they have been estrogen deficient for some time. This usually resolves by 3 months into treatment.

DURATION OF TREATMENT

Duration depends on the endpoints of treatment.

Vasomotor symptoms

Treatment for vasomotor symptoms should be continued for up to 5 years and then stopped to evaluate whether symptoms have recurred. Although most women do not experience menopausal symptoms after that time, some will flush into their 70s and even their 80s.

Prevention or treatment of osteoporosis

Treatment needs to be continued for life, as bone mineral density falls when treatment is stopped. Most epidemiological evidence suggests that 5–10 years of HRT soon after the menopause does not give any significant reduction in the risk of hip fracture 30 years later. Although some women will be happy to take HRT for life, others may view treatment as a continuum of options and will wish to change to other agents such as raloxifene, a bisphosphonate or strontium ranelate, because of the small increase in risk of breast cancer associated with the long-term use of combined HRT.

Premature menopause

Women usually are advised to continue with HRT until the average age of the natural menopause – that is, 52 years. Thereafter, the issues discussed in the above sections are relevant.

STOPPING HRT

Data to advise practice are limited. The limited evidence available shows no clear advantage of stopping gradually or abruptly. The main issue is a recurrence of menopausal symptoms, such as flushes and myalgia, and, as explained above, some women will flush into their 70s and 80s. There is no test which can predict which individual woman will flush. Anecdotally, older women need less estrogen to control their symptoms and, thus, doses can be gradually lowered. Although alternate-day or even less frequent oral treatment can be used in women who have had a hysterectomy, concerns exist that this strategy could lead to irregular bleeding or insufficient addition of progestogen in women whose uterus is intact. When systemic HRT is stopped, urogenital symptoms may become troublesome and topical estrogens can then be used (see Chapter 4).

MANAGING THE ADVERSE EFFECTS OF HRT

Adverse effects can be related to estrogen or progestogen, or a combination of both. Estrogen-related adverse effects include fluid retention, bloating, breast tenderness or enlargement, nausea, headaches, leg cramps and dyspepsia. Progestogen-related effects are fluid retention, breast tenderness, headaches or migraine, mood swings, depression, acne, lower abdominal pain and backache.

Adverse effects are usually transient and resolve without any change in treatment with increasing duration of use. Women should be encouraged to persist with therapy for about 12 weeks to await resolution. If symptoms persist beyond this, the options are:

- reduce the dose
- change estrogen/progestogen type
- change the route of delivery – oral to patch or gel, or intrauterine for progestogen
- change from sequential to continuous combined (but only in postmenopausal women).

ABNORMAL BLEEDING

Sequential regimens should produce regular predictable and acceptable bleeding, starting towards the end or soon after the end of the progestogen phase. However, withdrawal bleeds can be unacceptably heavy, prolonged or painful. Forgetting therapy, drug interactions (including with herbal remedies) or gastrointestinal upset, which can interfere with absorption, need to be excluded. Useful strategies include:

- increasing the dose or changing the type of progestogen
- considering intrauterine progestogen administration.

Pelvic pathology will need exclusion if the problem persists or does not respond to treatment (see Chapter 10). No bleeding reflects an atrophic endometrium and it occurs in 5% of women but pregnancy needs to be excluded in perimenopausal women.

Continuous combined regimens should result in no bleeding. However, breakthrough bleeding is common in the first 3–6 months of continuous combined therapy. If it continues thereafter, it should be investigated as for postmenopausal bleeding (see Chapter 10).

Further reading and sources of information

Archer DF, Hendrix S, Gallagher JC, Rymer J, Skouby S, Ferenczy A, *et al.* Endometrial effects of tibolone. *J Clin Endocrinol Metab* 2007;92:911–18.

British Menopause Society [www.thebms.org.uk].

Grady D, Sawaya GF. Discontinuation of postmenopausal hormone therapy. *Am J Med* 2005;118(Suppl 12B):163–5.

Kingsberg S. Testosterone treatment for hypoactive sexual desire disorder in postmenopausal women. *J Sex Med* 2007;4(Suppl 3):227–34.

North American Menopause Society. Role of progestogen in hormone therapy for postmenopausal women: position statement of the North American Menopause Society. *Menopause* 2003;10:113–32.

CKS. Clinical topic. Menopause [http://cks.library.nhs.uk/menopause].

Rees M, Purdie DW. *Management of the Menopause. The Handbook.* London: RSM Press; 2006.

4 Non-HRT options for osteoporosis

Several non-estrogen-based options are available for the prevention and treatment of osteoporosis (Table 6). Their use has mainly been evaluated in postmenopausal women with osteoporosis or at increased risk of the disease. There are few data in perimenopausal women (in their 50s)

Table 6   Interventions for the prevention and treatment of osteoporosis

	Spine	Hip
Bisphosphonates:		
Etidronate	A	B
Alendronate	A	A
Risedronate	A	A
Ibandronate	A	ND
Calcium and vitamin D	ND	A
Calcium	A	B
Calcitriol	A	ND
Calcitonin	A	B
Estrogen	A	A
SERMs	A	ND
Strontium ranelate	A	A
Parathyroid hormone peptides	A	ND

ND = not demonstrated

Levels of evidence:

A: meta-analysis of RCTs or from at least one RCT or from at least one well-designed controlled study without randomisation

B: from at least one other type of well-designed quasi-experimental study or from well-designed non-experimental descriptive studies, such as comparative studies, correlation studies, case–control studies or women with premature ovarian failure. There are concerns with agents such as bisphosphonates, which remain in bone for many years, on the fetal skeleton and they are not advised in women with fertility aspirations. Calcium and vitamin D supplements are considered in Chapter 6. Of note, these have been used in many studies in the placebo group.

Bisphosphonates

Bisphosphonates are chemical analogues of naturally occurring pyrophosphates, thus allowing them to be integrated into the skeleton. This makes metabolism an extremely slow process and the half-life of alendronate has been estimated to be as high as 12 years. Alendronate, risedronate, etidronate and ibandronate are used in the prevention and treatment of osteoporosis. The first three also are used in corticosteroid-induced osteoporosis.

Bisphosphonates can be classified into two groups:

- non-nitrogen-containing, such as etidronate
- nitrogen-containing, such as alendronate, risedronate and ibandronate.

All bisphosphonates are poorly absorbed and must be given on an empty stomach. Absorption is about 5–10% administered dose and can be inhibited by food or calcium-containing drinks (except water). The principal adverse effect of all bisphosphonates is upper gastrointestinal irritation. Thus, weekly and monthly regimens are preferred to daily dosing. Symptoms resolve quickly on stopping treatment.

The question of how long to prescribe a bisphosphonate has not been fully clarified yet, because of concerns about 'frozen bone', with complete turning off of bone remodelling with long-term use and also development of osteonecrosis in the jaw. Five years of treatment with a 2-year 'holiday' have been proposed for alendronate but differences may exist with individual bisphosphonates. This may not be applicable to glucocorticoid-induced osteoporosis.

The term osteonecrosis of the jaw is used to describe the exposure of bone within the oral cavity. Infection and dental extractions commonly precede presentation, although lesions can occur spontaneously. The vast majority of reports refer to high-dose intravenous bisphosphonates used in the oncological setting. Very few cases have been reported in women using oral bisphosphonates for osteoporosis. At this stage, clinical practice should not necessarily be altered but dental review could be considered in women with significant dental disease.

Comparisons have been made between alendronate and risedronate and between alendronate and raloxifene but, so far, they have been mainly limited to their effects on bone mineral density rather than the risk of fracture. Randomised controlled trials are awaited.

Alendronate

Alendronate reduces vertebral and non-vertebral fractures by 50% in RCTs. The dose for prevention of osteoporosis is 5 mg/day or 35 mg once weekly and for the treatment of established disease it is 10 mg/day or 70 mg once weekly.

Risedronate

Risedronate also reduces vertebral and non-vertebral fractures in RCTs. The dose for treatment of established disease is 5 mg/day or 35 mg once weekly.

Ibandronate

Ibandronate is an aminobisphosphonate that reduces vertebral but not non-vertebral fractures by 50% in RCTs undertaken in postmenopausal women. The dose is 2.5 mg/day or 150 mg once monthly orally or 3 mg intravenously every 3 months.

Etidronate

Etidronate was the first bisphosphonate to be developed and reduces the risk of vertebral but not non-vertebral fractures. It is given intermittently (400 mg on 14 of every 90 days) with 1250 mg of calcium carbonate (which, when dissolved in water, provides 500 mg of calcium as calcium citrate) during the remaining 76 days.

Strontium ranelate

Strontium is an alkaline earth element like calcium (group II in the periodic table) and is thus incorporated into the skeleton. RCTs have shown a decreased risk of vertebral and hip fractures with strontium ranelate. Oral absorption is poor but calcified tissues and areas of active osteogenesis take up 50–80% of the absorbed dose. The dose is a 2-g sachet/day and, like bisphosphonates, should be taken on an empty stomach. The most common adverse effects are mild and transient nausea and diarrhoea but are rare in absolute terms. A slight increase in the incidence of venous thromboembolism (0.9% compared with 0.6%) over 3 years was observed, without any underlying potential mechanism, as there is no known interaction between strontium ranelate and parameters of haemostasis. Strontium ranelate causes a clinically significant overestimation of bone mineral density because of the high attenuation of X-rays by strontium atoms in bone, as it has a higher atomic number than calcium (calcium 20, strontium 38). Corrections are being studied to allow interpretation of bone mineral density measurements in patients taking strontium ranelate.

Selective estrogen receptor modulators

Selective estrogen receptor modulators (SERMs) are compounds that possess estrogenic actions in certain tissues and anti-estrogenic actions in others. Tamoxifen was one of the first SERMs. As it behaves as an estrogen antagonist in the breast, it is used as an adjuvant treatment for breast cancer. It was also found to display beneficial estrogen agonist-like effects on bone and lipids but it has no licence for use in osteoporosis.

Raloxifene is licensed for the prevention of osteoporosis-related vertebral fracture. It reduces vertebral but not non-vertebral fracture by 30–50%, depending on the dose. The dose is 60 mg/day. It also reduces the risk of breast cancer to the same extent as tamoxifen. Adverse effects include hot flushes and calf cramps. It was thought that raloxifene could be cardio-protective from its effects on lipids but the Raloxifene Use for the Heart (RUTH) study found that it did not reduce the risk of coronary heart disease and it increased the risk of fatal stroke and venous thromboembolism. New SERMs such as bazedoxifene, arzoxifene, lasofoxifene and ospemifene are currently being evaluated.

Parathyroid hormone peptides

Although hyperparathyroidism is associated with bone loss, pulsed administration has the opposite effect. Recombinant 1-34 parathyroid hormone, given as a subcutaneous daily injection of 20 micrograms, reduces vertebral and non-vertebral fractures in postmenopausal women with osteoporosis. The full 1-84 parathyroid hormone peptide is given in the same way in a daily dose of 100 micrograms. They both reduce the risk of vertebral but not hip fractures. Because they cost more than other options, they are reserved for women with severe osteoporosis who are unable to tolerate or seem to be unresponsive to other treatments.

Calcitonin

Calcitonin can be given by subcutaneous or intramuscular injection or by nasal spray. Parenteral calcitonin is expensive, produces adverse effects such as nausea, diarrhoea and flushing and results in the production of neutralising antibodies in some patients. Nasal calcitonin also has been shown to reduce new vertebral fractures in women with established osteoporosis. Evidence exists for its efficacy as an analgesic in acute vertebral fracture. It also may be helpful as adjunctive treatment after surgery for hip fracture. An oral preparation is being developed.

Future developments

Annual intravenous administration of bisphosphonates is being studied.

Zoledronic acid is effective in reducing vertebral, hip and other fractures. Of concern is the fact that it may increase the risk of atrial fibrillation. Further data are awaited.

New therapeutic targets are being explored. Receptor activator of nuclear factor kappa B ligand (RANKL) is a cytokine member of the tumour necrosis factor family that is the principal final mediator of osteoclastic bone resorption. Denosumab (AMG 162) is an investigational fully human monoclonal antibody with a high affinity and specificity for RANKL. By inhibiting the action of RANKL, denosumab reduces the differentiation, activity and survival of osteoclasts, thereby slowing the rate of bone resorption. Denosumab has been shown to increase bone mineral density and reduce bone turnover in postmenopausal women with low bone mineral density.

Further reading

GENERAL

Keen R. Osteoporosis: strategies for prevention and management. *Best Pract Res Clin Rheumatol* 2007;21:109–22.

Lewiecki EM. RANK ligand inhibition with denosumab for the management of osteoporosis. *Expert Opin Biol Ther* 2006;6:1041–50.

Poole KE, Compston JE. Osteoporosis and its management. *BMJ* 2006;333:1251–6.

BISPHOSPHONATES

Basu N, Reid DM. Bisphosphonate-associated osteonecrosis of the jaw. *Menopause Int* 2007;13:56–9.

Black DM, Schwartz AV, Ensrud KE, Cauley JA, Levis S, Quandt SA, *et al;* FLEX Research Group. Effects of continuing or stopping alendronate after 5 years of treatment: the Fracture Intervention Trial Long-term Extension (FLEX): a randomized trial. *JAMA* 2006;296:2927–38.

Cooper C. Beyond daily dosing: clinical experience. *Bone* 2006;38(4 Suppl 1):S13–17.

Silverman SL, Watts NB, Delmas PD, Lange JL, Lindsay R. Effectiveness of bisphosphonates on nonvertebral and hip fractures in the first year of therapy: the risedronate and alendronate (REAL) cohort study. *Osteoporos Int* 2007;18:25–34.

Woo SB, Hande K, Richardson PG. Osteonecrosis of the jaw and bisphosphonates. *N Engl J Med* 2005;353:99–102.

STRONTIUM RANELATE

Roux C. Antifracture efficacy of strontium ranelate in postmenopausal osteoporosis. *Bone* 2007;40(5 Suppl 1):S9–11.

Blake GM, Fogelman I. Effect of bone strontium on BMD measurements. *J Clin Densitom* 2007;10:34–8.

O'Donnell S, Cranney A, Wells GA, Adachi JD, Reginster JY. Strontium ranelate for preventing and treating postmenopausal osteoporosis. *Cochrane Database Syst Rev* 2006;3:CD005326.

SELECTIVE ESTROGEN RECEPTOR MODULATORS

Barrett-Connor E, Mosca L, Collins P, Geiger MJ, Grady D, Kornitzer M, *et al;* Raloxifene Use for The Heart (RUTH) Trial Investigators. Effects of raloxifene on cardiovascular events and breast cancer in postmenopausal women. *N Engl J Med* 2006;355:125–37.

Palacios S. The future of the new selective estrogen receptor modulators. *Menopause Int* 2007;13:27–34.

Vogel VG, Costantino JP, Wickerham DL, Cronin WM, Cecchini RS, Atkins JN, *et al;* National Surgical Adjuvant Breast and Bowel Project (NSABP). Effects of tamoxifen vs raloxifene on the risk of developing invasive breast cancer and other disease outcomes: the NSABP Study of Tamoxifen and Raloxifene (STAR) P-2 trial. *JAMA* 2006;295:2727–41.

PARATHYROID HORMONE PEPTIDES

Greenspan SL, Bone HG, Ettinger MP, Hanley DA, Lindsay R, Zanchetta JR, *et al;* Treatment of Osteoporosis with Parathyroid Hormone Study Group. Effect of recombinant human parathyroid hormone (1-84) on vertebral fracture and bone mineral density in postmenopausal women with osteoporosis: a randomized trial. *Ann Intern Med* 2007;146:326–39.

Neer RM, Arnaud CD, Zanchetta JR, Prince R, Gaich GA, Reginster JY, *et al.* Effect of parathyroid hormone on vertebral bone mass and fracture incidence among postmenopausal women with osteoporosis. *N Engl J Med* 2001;344:1434–41.

CALCITONIN

Knopp JA, Diner BM, Blitz M, Lyritis GP, Rowe BH. Calcitonin for treating acute pain of osteoporotic vertebral compression fractures: a systematic review of randomized, controlled trials. *Osteoporos Int* 2005;16:1281–90.

Munoz-Torres M, Alonso G, Raya MP. Calcitonin therapy in osteoporosis. *Treat Endocrinol* 2004;3:117–32.

FUTURE DEVELOPMENTS

Black DM, Delmas PD, Eastell R, Reid IR, Boonen S, Cauley JA, *et al;* HORIZON Pivotal Fracture Trial. Once-yearly zoledronic acid for treatment of postmenopausal osteoporosis. *N Engl J Med* 2007;356:1809–22.

Lyles KW, Colon-Emeric CS, Magaziner JS, Adachi JD, Pieper CF, Mautalen C, *et al;* HORIZON Recurrent Fracture Trial. Zoledronic acid and clinical fractures and mortality after hip fracture. *N Engl J Med* 2007;357:1799–809.

McClung M. Role of RANKL inhibition in osteoporosis. *Arthritis Res Ther* 2007;9 Suppl 1:S3.

5   Diet and lifestyle

This chapter examines diet, exercise, smoking cessation and weight loss. Notwithstanding the obesity epidemic, undernutrition in the elderly is a significant medical problem. It leads to the 'anorexia of ageing' and is associated with increased morbidity and mortality. The nutritional requirements of older women are of increasing interest as more are living into their 80s and beyond. Exercise needs to be promoted and continued, as it maintains muscle and bone mass and thus prevents falls and osteoporotic fractures.

Diet

Dietary components can be classified into macronutrients, micronutrients and functional foods.

MACRONUTRIENTS

Macronutrients encompass carbohydrate, protein and fat.

Carbohydrate
The World Health Organization has recommended that 55–75% of energy input should come from carbohydrate, with less than 10% from free sugars. The proportion coming from non-milk extrinsic sugars, from foods such as sugar and preserves, is important. Diets high in non-milk extrinsic sugars may reduce intake of foods that are more nutrient dense. More emphasis is needed on other carbohydrate-rich foods (such as wholegrain breakfast cereals, grains and breads), which also provide fibre and some B vitamins.

Protein
Current recommendations are 10–15% of total energy intake. As lean body mass decreases with age, protein requirements increase to maintain nitrogen equilibrium. Demand further increases in wound healing (including fractures), infection and restoring muscle mass lost from immobility.

Fat

The World Health Organization has recommended that total fat intake should account for 15–30% of total energy intake, with saturated fats accounting for less than 10% and polyunsaturated fats for 6–10%. The Women's Health Initiative RCT examined the effect of reduction of total fat intake on the risk of breast and colorectal cancer and cardiovascular disease. In this study, 16 541 women were assigned to a diet with reduced total fat intake (20% total energy) and increased intakes of vegetables, fruits and grains. The comparison group of 29 294 women did not have any dietary changes and mean follow-up was 8.1 years. The dietary intervention had no effect.

Particular types, such as omega 3 fatty acids that are found mainly in oily fish, may be important. Much of the interest in the association between omega 3 fatty acids and cardiovascular disease follows studies with Greenland Inuit people, who traditionally have low mortality from coronary heart disease despite a diet rich in fat. A systematic review has found no cardiovascular benefit but this observation may reflect the characteristics of the populations in the included trials. On the other hand, seafood intake may protect against Alzheimer's disease and dementia and this protection may be mediated by omega 3 fatty acids.

MICRONUTRIENTS

Micronutrients encompass vitamins and minerals. Low levels of calcium and vitamin D are associated with poor skeletal health and osteoporotic fractures. There are claims that antioxidant supplements are associated with reduced mortality. It has been estimated that 10–20% of the adult population (80–160 million people) in North America and Europe may take antioxidants with claims that they improve health. However, a meta-analysis has shown that while beta carotene, vitamin A and vitamin E increased mortality, vitamin C and selenium did not appear to have a significant effect. There was no convincing evidence that antioxidant supplements have beneficial effects on mortality. These findings with synthetic antioxidants should not be extrapolated to potential effects of fruits and vegetables, which contain other substances such as fibre and flavonoids.

Vitamin A is important for normal vision, cell differentiation, immune function and genetic expression. Of note is the fact that a high vitamin A intake is associated with a higher risk for fractures as it is a vitamin D and calcium antagonist.

Calcium and vitamin D

Supplementation with calcium and vitamin D, particularly, may be

BOX 3. CALCIUM CONTENT OF SOME FOODS	
Food	**Calcium content (mg)**
Full-fat milk (250 ml)	295
Semi-skimmed milk (250 ml)	300
Skimmed milk (250 ml)	305
Low-fat yogurt (100 g)	150
Cheddar cheese (50 g)	360
Boiled spinach (100 g)	159
Brazil nuts (100 g)	170
Tinned salmon (100 g)	93
Tofu (100 g)	480

relevant when evidence of insufficiency exists. Provision of adequate dietary or supplemental calcium and vitamin D is an essential part of the management of osteoporosis. In northern latitudes, cutaneous synthesis of vitamin D occurs only in the summer months and many diets lack sufficient amounts of this vitamin for adequate intake in the absence of solar exposure. Some countries, such as the USA, fortify foods by adding vitamin D to dairy products.

The calcium content of some foods is shown in Box 3. Most studies show that about 1.5 g of elemental calcium is necessary to preserve bone health in postmenopausal women and elderly women who are not taking HRT. This figure has been reinforced by the US National Institutes of Health. The effects of calcium and vitamin D supplements alone or in combination on fracture, however, are contradictory and may depend on the study population. For example, people in sheltered accommodation or residential care may be more frail, may have lower dietary intakes of calcium and vitamin D and are at higher risk of fracture than those living in the community. While an early study of institutionalised women showed benefit, this has not been consistently found in community dwelling women or as secondary prevention. Benefits are greater when compliance rates are higher. As a note of caution, the WHI study showed an increase in kidney stones in women at low risk of stones who were taking calcium and vitamin D supplements.

Calcitriol is the active metabolite of vitamin D which facilitates the intestinal absorption of calcium. It also has direct effects on bone cells. Studies of the effects of calcitriol on bone loss and fractures have produced conflicting results. The potential dangers of hypercalcaemia and hypercalciuria mean that levels of calcium in serum and urine should be monitored closely, so limiting its use.

Vitamin B12 and folate

Vitamin B12 (cobolamin) and folate deficiency may lead to macrocytic anaemia and neurological problems. Vitamins E and C protect the body from damage from free radicals. However, supplements do not reduce mortality (see above).

FUNCTIONAL FOODS

Functional foods generally are defined as foods that confer a 'benefit' to the host beyond simple nutrition. Five main types of functional foods may be important in women's health:

- probiotics
- prebiotics
- synbiotics
- nutraceuticals
- fibre.

Probiotics are defined as a 'live microbial feed supplement which beneficially affects the host animal by improving its intestinal balance'. Currently, the best-studied probiotics are the lactic acid bacteria, particularly *Lactobacillus spp.* and *Bifidobacterium spp.* These can be combined with food products such as cereals, bioyoghurts and drinks. Increasing evidence shows the potential of probiotics in benefiting gastrointestinal conditions (such as diarrhoea and irritable bowel syndrome) and non-gastrointestinal tract conditions (such as candidiasis and urinary tract infections).

Prebiotics are 'non-digestible food ingredients which selectively stimulate a limited number of bacteria in the colon, to improve host health'. The emphasis of prebiotic research is to enhance the indigenous probiotic flora. This includes strategies to develop specific prebiotics for individual probiotic organisms, as well as aiding persistence of prebiotic effects throughout the gastrointestinal tract. They may be involved in calcium absorption.

Synbiotics contain complementary pro- and prebiotics that interact to provide a synergistic effect towards the maintenance of a desirable microbial population in the intestinal microbiota.

Nutraceuticals are natural components of foods (such as isoflavones and phytoestrogens) that may be released during digestion and therefore become bioavailable (see Chapter 6).

Fibre consists of plant substances that resist hydrolysis by digestive enzymes in the small bowel. Fibre can be classified according to its solubility and fermentability by bacteria: a soluble fibre is readily fermentable by colonic bacteria and an insoluble fibre only slowly fermentable. Fibre may lower serum cholesterol and improve glycaemic control.

THE MEDITERRANEAN DIET

The Mediterranean diet is compatible with healthier ageing and increased longevity. It may also lower the risk of Alzheimer's disease. The Mediterranean diet is characterised by a high intake of vegetables, legumes, fruits and cereals (in the past largely unrefined); a moderate to high intake of fish; a low intake of saturated lipids but a high intake of unsaturated lipids, particularly olive oil; a low to moderate intake of dairy products, mostly cheese and yogurt; a low intake of meat; and a modest intake of alcohol, mostly as wine. Mediterranean and modified Mediterranean diets are associated with reductions in mortality.

FLAVONOIDS

Flavonoids are polyphenolic compounds found in small quantities in numerous plant foods, including fruit and vegetables, tea, wine, nuts and seeds, herbs and spices. There has been increasing interest due to growing evidence of their versatile health benefits such as reducing risk of cardio-vascular disease and cancer.

Exercise

Regular physical activity for postmenopausal women reduces the risk of falls, osteoporotic fractures, CHD and type-2 diabetes mellitus. Furthermore, hot flushes also may be improved by physical activity but the evidence is conflicting. Exercise methods can be divided into three general categories:

- endurance exercise
- strength exercise
- balance exercise
- vibration exercise.

EXERCISE AND THE SKELETON

The role of exercise in preventing osteoporotic fractures is well established; however, what types, intensity, frequency and duration of activity are most effective is unclear. Physical activity is not only an important determinant of peak bone mass but also helps to maintain bone mass in later life. A Cochrane review found that fast walking effectively improved bone density in the spine and the hip, whereas weight-bearing exercises were associated with increases in bone density of the spine but not the hip. Exercise regimens can be very helpful in the management of established osteoporosis. The benefits are mainly related to increased wellbeing, muscle strength, postural stability and a reduction of chronic pain, rather than an increase of skeletal mass. Exercise has to be structured carefully because of concerns about falls and fractures. Vibration exercise is a new modality, initially studied in athletes, that is being explored in the elderly.

EXERCISE AND THE HEART

Exercise has a direct effect on the cardiovascular system by increasing oxygen delivery and use, reducing the progression of atherosclerosis and by decreasing the risk of ventricular arrhythmias and the overall risk of sudden cardiac death. In addition, physical activity can increase levels of high-density lipoprotein cholesterol. The indirect effects of exercise such as reductions in body weight, may also be important. The optimal type, frequency and intensity are uncertain. Low-intensity exercise, such as walking (with which fewer concerns about falls exist), can reduce the risk of cardiovascular disease to a degree similar to that achieved with more vigorous physical activity.

Smoking cessation

Smoking related-diseases kill one in ten adults globally or cause four million deaths. Smoking reduces life expectancy and increases the risk of cardiovascular disease, cancer, chronic obstructive pulmonary disease and dementia. It also increases the overall lifetime risk of a woman developing a vertebral or hip fracture by 13% and 31%, respectively. Clearly, there are many reasons why smoking should be discouraged.

Weight reduction

Women gain weight with age, and this tends to begin at or near menopause. Weight gain is in the region of 2 kg. Body fat distribution also changes independent of weight gain, again starting around the time of the menopause. There is an increase in body fat as a percentage of body weight and a redistribution of body fat, with a relative increase in the proportion of abdominal fat. This centralised abdominal (android) fat distribution is a recognised risk factor for cardiovascular disease.

The reasons why women gain weight are disputed. However, regular physical activity may reduce weight gain and the adverse changes in body composition and fat distribution that accompany ageing and the menopausal transition.

A Health Technology Assessment review of obesity treatments modelled the impact of weight reduction on risk factor change. Women with obesity-related diseases, who had intentional weight loss, had an associated reduced risk of death, cardiovascular disease death, cancer and diabetes-related death. However, it not currently known whether weight loss improves health outcomes in postmenopausal women, since most studies are short, being about 12 months in duration.

Further reading

DIET

Barberger-Gateau P, Letenneur L, Deschamps V, Pérès K, Dartigues JF, Renaud S. Fish, meat, and risk of dementia: cohort study. *BMJ* 2002;325:932–3.

Beresford SA, Johnson KC, Ritenbaugh C, Lasser NL, Snetselaar LG, Black HR, *et al.* Low-fat dietary pattern and risk of colorectal cancer: the Women's Health Initiative randomized controlled dietary modification trial. *JAMA* 2006;295:643–54.

Bischoff-Ferrari HA, Willett WC, Wong JB, Giovannucci E, Dietrich T, Dawson-Hughes B. Fracture prevention with vitamin D supplementation: a meta-analysis of randomized controlled trials. *JAMA* 2005;293:2257–64.

Bjelakovic G, Nikolova D, Gluud LL, Simonetti RG, Gluud C. Mortality in randomized trials of antioxidant supplements for primary and secondary prevention: systematic review and meta-analysis. *JAMA* 2007;297:842–57.

Din JN, Newby DE, Flapan AD. Omega 3 fatty acids and cardiovascular disease: fishing for a natural treatment. *BMJ* 2004;328:30–5.

Grant AM, Avenell A, Campbell MK, McDonald AM, MacLennan GS, McPherson GC, *et al.* Oral vitamin D3 and calcium for secondary prevention of low-trauma fractures in elderly people (Randomised Evaluation of Calcium Or vitamin D, RECORD): a randomised placebo-controlled trial. *Lancet* 2005;365:1621–8.

Hooper L, Thompson RL, Harrison RA, Summerbell CD, Ness AR, Moore HJ, *et al.* Risks and benefits of omega3 fats for mortality, cardiovascular disease and cancer: a systematic review. *BMJ* 2006;332:752–5.

Howard BV, Van Horn L, Hsia J, Manson JE, Stefanick ML, Wassertheil-Smoller S, *et al.* Low-fat dietary pattern and risk of cardiovascular disease: the Women's Health Initiative Randomized Controlled Dietary Modification Trial. *JAMA* 2006;295:655–66.

Jackson RD, LaCroix AZ, Gass M, Wallace RB, Robbins J, Lewis CE, *et al*; Women's Health Initiative Investigators. Calcium plus vitamin D supplementation and the risk of fractures. *N Engl J Med* 2006;354:669–83.

Mink PJ, Scrafford CG, Barraj LM, Harnack L, Hong CP, Nettleton JA, *et al.* Flavonoid intake and cardiovascular disease mortality: a prospective study in postmenopausal women. *Am J Clin Nutr* 2007;85:895–909.

Morris MC, Evans DA, Tangney CC, Bienias JL, Wilson RS. Fish consumption and cognitive decline with age in a large community study. *Arch Neurol* 2005;62:1849–53.

Porthouse J, Cockayne S, King C, Saxon L, Steele E, Aspray T, *et al.* Randomised controlled trial of calcium and supplementation with cholecalciferol (vitamin D3) for prevention of fractures in primary care. *BMJ* 2005;330:1003–6.

Prentice RL, Thomson CA, Caan B, Hubbell FA, Anderson GL, Beresford SA, *et al.* Low-fat dietary pattern and risk of invasive breast cancer: the Women's Health Initiative Randomized Controlled Dietary Modification Trial. *JAMA* 2006;295:629–42.

Prince RL. Calcium and vitamin D: for whom and when. *Menopause Int* 2007;13:35–7.

National Institutes of Health. Optimal Calcium Intake. Consensus Development Conference Statement June 6–8, 1994 [http://consensus.nih.gov/1994/1994OptimalCalcium097html.htm].

Reginster JY. The high prevalence of inadequate serum vitamin D levels and implications for bone health. *Curr Med Res Opin* 2005;21:579–86.

Serra-Majem L, Roman B, Estruch R. Scientific evidence of interventions using the Mediterranean diet: a systematic review. *Nutr Rev* 2006;64:S27–47.

Shea B, Wells G, Cranney A, Zytaruk N, Robinson V, Griffith L, *et al.* Calcium supplementation on bone loss in postmenopausal women. *Cochrane Database Syst Rev* 2004;(1):CD004526.

Smejkal C. Functional foods. In: Rees M, Mander T, editors. *Managing the Menopause Without Oestrogen.* London: RSM Press; 2004.

Tang BM, Eslick GD, Nowson C, Smith C, Bensoussan A.Use of calcium or calcium in combination with vitamin D supplementation to prevent fractures and bone loss in people aged 50 years and older: a meta-analysis. *Lancet* 2007;370:657–66.

Trichopoulou A, Critselis E. Mediterranean diet and longevity. *Eur J Cancer Prev* 2004;13:453–6.

Diet, nutrition and the prevention of chronic diseases. Report of the joint WHO/FAO expert consultation. *World Health Organ Tech Rep Ser* 2003;916: i–viii, 1–149 [www.who.int/dietphysicalactivity/publications/trs916/en/].

Yao LH, Jiang YM, Shi J, Tomás-Barberán FA, Datta N, Singanusong R, *et al.* Flavonoids in food and their health benefits. *Plant Foods Hum Nutr* 2004;59:113–22.

EXERCISE

Asikainen TM, Kukkonen-Harjula K, Miilunpalo S. Exercise for health for early postmenopausal women: a systematic review of randomised controlled trials. *Sports Med* 2004;34:753–78.

Bonaiuti D, Shea B, Iovine R, Negrini S, Robinson V, Kemper HC, *et al.* Exercise for preventing and treating osteoporosis in postmenopausal women. *Cochrane Database Syst Rev* 2003;(4):CD0000333.

Cardinale M, Rittweger J. Vibration exercise makes your muscles and bones stronger: fact or fiction? *J Br Menopause Soc* 2006;12:12–18.

Lindh-Astrand L, Nedstrand E, Wyon Y, Hammar M. Vasomotor symptoms and quality of life in previously sedentary postmenopausal women randomised to physical activity or estrogen therapy. *Maturitas* 2004;48:97–105.

Manson JE, Greenland P, LaCroix AZ, Stefanick ML, Mouton CP, Oberman A, *et al.* Walking compared with vigorous exercise for the prevention of cardiovascular events in women. *N Engl J Med* 2002;347:716–25.

Wayne PM, Kiel DP, Krebs DE, Davis RB, Savetsky-German J, Connelly M, *et al.* The effects of Tai Chi on bone mineral density in postmenopausal women: a systematic review. *Arch Phys Med Rehabil* 2007;88:673–80.

SMOKING CESSATION AND WEIGHT REDUCTION

Aggarwal NT, Bienias JL, Bennett DA, Wilson RS, Morris MC, Schneider JA, *et al.* The relation of cigarette smoking to incident Alzheimer's disease in a biracial urban community population. *Neuroepidemiology* 2006;26:140–6.

Avenell A, Broom J, Brown TJ, Poobalan A, Aucott L, Stearns SC, *et al.* Systematic review of the long-term consequences of treatments for obesity and implications for health improvement. *Health Technol Assess* 2004;8:iii-iv, 1–182.

Brown TJ. Health benefits of weight reduction in postmenopausal women: a systematic review. *J Br Menopause Soc* 2006;12:164–71.

Gill JM, Malkova D. Physical activity, fitness and cardiovascular disease risk in adults: interactions with insulin resistance and obesity. *Clin Sci (Lond)* 2006;110:409–25.

Sternfeld B, Bhat AK, Wang H, Sharp T, Quesenberry CP Jr. Menopause, physical activity, and body composition/fat distribution in midlife women. *Med Sci Sports Exerc* 2005;37:1195–202.

Sternfeld B, Wang H, Quesenberry CP Jr, Abrams B, Everson-Rose SA, Greendale GA, *et al.* Physical activity and changes in weight and waist circumference in midlife women: findings from the Study of Women's Health Across the Nation. *Am J Epidemiol* 2004;160:912–22.

Ward KD, Klesges RC. A meta-analysis of the effects of cigarette smoking on bone mineral density. *Calcif Tissue Int* 2001;68:259–70.

Williams LT, Young AF, Brown WJ. Weight gained in two years by a population of mid-aged women: how much is too much? *Int J Obes (Lond)* 2006;30:1229–33.

World Health Organization. Smoking statistics [www.wpro.who.int/media_centre/fact_sheets/fs_20020528.htm].

6 Alternative and complementary therapies

Concerns about the safety of estrogen-based HRT after publication of the Women's Health Initiative study and Million Women Study have led to women turning to alternative and complementary therapies erroneously believing that they are safer and 'more natural'. In the USA, one in three adults uses such strategies and, worryingly, may not consult their health professional. There are major concerns about interactions with other treatments, with potentially fatal consequences. Concern also exists about the quality control of production and contaminants such as arsenic, lead or mercury. While a European Union Directive on traditional herbal medicinal products was implemented in October 2005 in the UK, this will not cover products bought by women outside Europe. Evidence from randomised trials that alternative and complementary and therapies improve menopausal symptoms or have the same benefits as conventional pharmacopoeia is poor.

Herbal products

A wide variety of herbs are used and a summary regarding their efficacy and safety is given below.

ACTAEA RACEMOSA (BLACK COHOSH)

The root and rhizome of black cohosh, an indigenous North American herb, have been extensively researched for the relief of menopause-related symptoms. German health authorities endorse the use of black cohosh extract for premenstrual discomfort, dysmenorrhea and menopause. Similarly, the World Health Organization recognises its use for 'treatment of climacteric symptoms such as hot flushes, profuse sweating, sleeping disorders and nervous irritability'. Most studies indicate that black cohosh extract reduces some symptoms associated with menopause; however, methodologic shortcomings and variations in product and dosage limit definitive conclusions. Also, the wide variety of black cohosh products and formulations make comparisons between clinical trials difficult. While it may act via nonhormonal mechanisms, it may have estrogenic actions leading to concerns about its use in women with breast cancer. There have also been reports of liver toxicity.

ANGELICA SINENSIS (DONG QUAI)

Dong quai root has been used to treat a variety of disorders in traditional Chinese medicine for many centuries. It was not found to be superior to placebo in a randomised trial. Interaction with warfarin and photosensitisation have been reported.

OENOTHERA BIENNIS (EVENING PRIMROSE)

Evening primrose oil is extracted from the seeds of the evening primrose plant, a wildflower native to North America. The seed oil is a rich source of linoleic acid and gamma linolenic acid. One small, placebo-controlled, randomised trial showed it to be ineffective for treating hot flushes.

PANAX GINSENG (GINSENG)

Ginseng root has held a place of importance in Asian medicine for millennia. As the common name, ginseng, is used to describe a number of chemically different species of *Panax*, caution must be exercised when interpreting data between species. German health authorities and the WHO endorse the use of *Panax ginseng* as a tonic or restorative agent for invigoration and fortification in times of fatigue, debility, or physical or mental exhaustion. It was not found to be superior to placebo for menopausal symptoms in a randomised trial. Case reports have associated ginseng with postmenopausal bleeding and mastalgia. Interactions have been observed with warfarin, phenelzine and alcohol.

PIPER METHYSTICUM (KAVA KAVA)

In the South Pacific, kava kava has been used for recreational and medicinal purposes for thousands of years. A Cochrane review concluded that it may be an effective symptomatic treatment for anxiety but the data about menopausal symptoms are conflicting. Concern about liver damage has led regulatory authorities to suspend or withdraw kava kava.

GINKGO BILOBA (GINGKO)

The use of *Gingko biloba* is widespread but little evidence shows that it improves menopausal symptoms.

OTHER HERBS

Wild yam cream, dong quai, *Hypericum perforatum* (St John's wort), *Agnus castus* (chasteberry), liquorice root and valerian root also are popular but no good evidence shows that they have any effect on menopausal symptoms. Claims have been made that steroids (diosgenein) in yams (*Dioscorea villosa*) can be converted in the body to progesterone but this is biochemically impossible in humans.

Herb–drug interactions

A major concern about herbs is herb–drug interactions with potentially fatal consequences as well as estrogenic effects, which is important in women with hormone-dependent tumours. The consequences of herb–drug interactions include bleeding when combined with warfarin or aspirin; hypertension, coma and mild serotonin syndrome when combined with serotonin reuptake inhibitors; and reduced efficacy of antiepileptics and oral contraceptives. For example, *Ginkgo biloba* can cause bleeding when combined with warfarin or aspirin, high blood pressure when combined with a thiazide diuretic and even coma when combined with trazodone. *Panax ginseng* reduces the blood concentrations of alcohol and warfarin and can induce mania when used concomitantly with phenelzine. *Hypericum perforatum* reduces the blood concentrations of cyclosporin, midazolam, tacrolimus, amitriptyline, digoxin, warfarin and theophylline. Reduced concentrations of cyclosporin have led to organ rejection. *Hypericum* also causes breakthrough bleeding and unplanned pregnancies when used concomitantly with oral contraceptives. It also causes serotonin syndrome when used in combination with selective serotonin reuptake inhibitors (for example, sertraline and paroxetine). Furthermore, little control over the quality of the products exists, so it is unusual to know what is actually present in individual herbal preparations and dietary supplements. Severe adverse reactions, including renal and liver failure and cancer, have been reported.

Phytoestrogens: soy and red clover

Phytoestrogens are plant substances that have effects similar to those of estrogens. The most important groups are called isoflavones and lignans. The major isoflavones are genistein and daidzein. The major lignans are enterolactone and enterodiol. Isoflavones are found in soybeans, chickpeas, red clover and probably other legumes (beans and peas). Oilseeds such as flaxseed are rich in lignans and they also are found in cereal bran, whole cereals, vegetables, legumes and fruit. It has been postulated that dietary intake of soy may explain, in part, the lower reporting of hot flushes by Asian women. Populations that consume a diet high in phytoestrogens are said to have lower rates of cardiovascular disease, osteoporosis and breast, colon, endometrial and ovarian cancers. Phytos, Isoheart and Phytoprevent are European Union studies examining the role of phytoestrogens in osteoporosis, heart disease and cancer. Further well-designed, randomised trials are needed to determine the role and safety of phytoestrogen supplements in menopausal women and cancer survivors.

Soy

The results from clinical trials are contradictory and difficult to evaluate owing to variation in soy preparations, dosages and durations of treatment. Furthermore, substantial inter-individual differences in isoflavone metabolism exist in the general population, which may also affect study outcomes. The isoflavone daidzein is metabolised extensively in the gut to the more estrogenic secondary metabolite equol by the human gut microflora. That only 30% of Western populations excrete high levels of equol might account for the conflicting evidence provided by clinical trials.

Soy extracts appear to be well tolerated, with few if any serious adverse effects noted in clinical studies. However, endometrial hyperplasia has been reported in soy users.

Red clover

Although red clover blossoms have been used in traditional herbal medicine for centuries, it is the semi-purified isoflavone leaf extracts for relief of menopause-related symptoms that interest researchers. Clinical trials for menopause-related symptoms have been conducted primarily with the proprietary semi-purified isoflavone leaf extracts. The majority of clinical data do not support the efficacy of semi-purified isoflavone red clover leaf extracts in reducing hot flush frequency and severity. No serious adverse effect has been reported in clinical trials or in the medical literature but because red clover leaf extracts contain semi-purified isoflavones, the question of safety in hormone-sensitive tissue is important. At present, the safety of red clover leaf extracts in women with a history of breast cancer is unknown.

Homoeopathy

Homoeopathy aims to treat 'like with like' and the term 'homoeopathy' was coined by the German physician, Christian Friedrich Samuel Hahnemann (1755–1843). Homoeopathic remedies are extremely diluted agents. Adherents and practitioners of homoeopathy assert that the therapeutic potency of a remedy can be increased by serial dilution of the drug, combined with succussion or vigorous shaking. This dilution is often repeated such that there is no active molecule present in the solution. Homeopathy regards diseases as morbid derangements of the organism and states that instances of disease in different people differ fundamentally. Homoeopathy views a sick person as having a dynamic disturbance in a hypothetical 'vital force', a disturbance which, homoeopaths claim, underlies standard medical diagnoses of named diseases. The mechanisms that underlie the biological response to ultramolecular dilutions, however, are scientifically unclear. Homoeopathy has received criticisms on theoretical grounds. Data from case histories, observational studies and a small number of randomised trials are encouraging but more research clearly is needed.

Dehydroepiandrosterone

Dehydroepiandrosterone (DHEA) is a steroid secreted by the adrenal cortex. It mostly is produced in a sulphated form (DHEA-S), which may be converted to DHEA in many tissues. Blood levels of DHEA decrease dramatically with age. This led to suggestions that the effects of ageing can be counteracted by DHEA 'replacement therapy'. Dehydroepiandrosterone is marketed as a food supplement in the USA, for its supposed anti-ageing effects. There is currently no evidence that DHEA has any effect on hot flushes. Safety is unknown.

Progesterone transdermal creams

Progesterone has been prepared in gels and creams for a number of years. One licensed gel is available in Europe; however, it is indicated for local use on the breast but not for systemic therapy. A vaginal gel for endometrial protection has been studied.

Progesterone transdermal creams have been advocated for the treatment of menopausal symptoms and skeletal protection. They contain micronised progesterone. At present, there are insufficient published data that transdermal progesterone reduces hot flushes or protects the skeleton. Similarly, transdermal progesterone creams cannot prevent mitotic activity or induce secretory change in an estrogen-primed endometrium. Thus, women who use systemic estrogen and transdermal progesterone creams are increasing their risk of endometrial cancer. Again further research is needed.

Physical therapies

The term 'physical' is used, as these therapies do not involve ingestion or application of any agent. These include acupuncture, reflexology, acupressure, Alexander technique, Ayurveda, osteopathy, magnetism and Reiki. There is very little evidence that they help menopausal symptoms.

Further reading

Balk E, Chung M, Chew P, Ip S, Raman G, Kupelnick B, *et al.* Effects of soy on health outcomes. *Evid Rep Technol Assess (Summ)* 2005;126:1–8.

British Menopause Society Council Consensus Statement 2007 Alternative and Complementary Therapies [www.thebms.org.uk/statementcontent.php?id=2].

Carpenter JS, Neal JG. Other complementary and alternative medicine modalities: acupuncture, magnets, reflexology, and homeopathy. *Am J Med* 2005;118(Suppl 12B):109–17.

De Smet PA. Clinical risk management of herb-drug interactions. *Br J Clin Pharmacol* 2007;63:258–67.

Dodin S, Lemay A, Jacques H, Légaré F, Forest JC, Mâsse B.The effects of flaxseed dietary supplement on lipid profile, bone mineral density, and symptoms in menopausal women: a randomized, double-blind, wheat germ placebo-controlled clinical trial. *J Clin Endocrinol Metab* 2005;90:1390–7.

Garvey GJ, Hahn G, Lee RV, Harbison RD. Heavy metal hazards of Asian traditional remedies. *Int J Environ Health Res* 2001;11:63–71.

Hinson J, Raven P. Dehydroepiandrosterone (DHEA) and the menopause: an update. *Menopause Int* 2007;13(2):75–8.

Howes LG, Howes JB, Knight DC. Isoflavone therapy for menopausal flushes: a systematic review and meta-analysis. *Maturitas* 2006;55:203–11.

Hu Z, Yang X, Ho PC, Chan SY, Heng PW, Chan E, *et al.* Herb-drug interactions: a literature review. *Drugs* 2005;65:1239–82.

Loudon I. A brief history of homeopathy. *J R Soc Med* 2006;99:607–10.

Low Dog T. Menopause: a review of botanical dietary supplements. *Am J Med* 2005;118(Suppl 12B):98–108.

Medicines and Healthcare products Regulatory Agency. Traditional Herbal Medicine Registration Scheme [www.mhra.gov.uk/home/].

Messina M, McCaskill-Stevens W, Lampe JW. Addressing the soy and breast cancer relationship: review, commentary, and workshop proceedings. *J Natl Cancer Inst* 2006;98:1275–84.

Meijerman I, Beijnen JH, Schellens JH. Herb–drug interactions in oncology: focus on mechanisms of induction. *Oncologist* 2006;11:742–52.

Nedrow A, Miller J, Walker M, Nygren P, Huffman LH, Nelson HD. Complementary and alternative therapies for the management of menopause-related symptoms: a systematic evidence review. *Arch Intern Med* 2006;166:1453–65.

Newton KM, Reed SD, LaCroix AZ, Grothaus LC, Ehrlich K, Guiltinan J. Treatment of vasomotor symptoms of menopause with black cohosh, multibotanicals, soy, hormone therapy, or placebo: a randomized trial. *Ann Intern Med* 2006;145:869–79.

Royal College and Obstetricians and Gynaecologists. *Alternatives to HRT for the Management of Symptoms of the Menopause.* Scientific Advisory Committee Opinion Paper 6. London: RCOG; 2006 [www.rcog.org.uk/index.asp?PageID=1561].

Taylor DM, Walsham N, Taylor SE, Wong L. Potential interactions between prescription drugs and complementary and alternative medicines among patients in the emergency department. *Pharmacotherapy* 2006;26:634–40.

Tice JA, Ettinger B, Ensrud K, Wallace R, Blackwell T, Cummings SR. Phytoestrogen supplements for the treatment of hot flashes: the Isoflavone Clover Extract (ICE) Study: a randomized controlled trial. *JAMA* 2003;290:207–14.

Tindle HA, Davis RB, Phillips RS, Eisenberg DM. Trends in use of complementary and alternative medicine by US adults: 1997–2002. *Altern Ther Health Med* 2005;11:42–9.

Van de Weijer PHM, Barentsen R. Isoflavones from red clover (Promensil®) significantly reduce menopausal hot flush symptoms compared with placebo. *Maturitas* 2002;42:187–93.

Vashisht A, Wadsworth F, Carey A, Carey B, Studd J. Bleeding profiles and effects on the endometrium for women using a novel combination of transdermal oestradiol and natural progesterone cream as part of a continuous combined hormone replacement regime. *BJOG* 2005;112:1402–6.

Wren BG, Champion SM, Willetts K, Manga RZ, Eden JA. Transdermal progesterone and its effect on vasomotor symptoms, blood lipid levels, bone metabolic markers, moods, and quality of life for postmenopausal women. *Menopause* 2003;10:13–18

7 Vasomotor symptoms, urogenital and sexual problems

Vasomotor symptoms

Hot flushes and night sweats are the most common symptoms of the menopause and these affect about 70% of Western women. Night sweats can also cause profound sleep disturbance leading to tiredness and irritability. They may begin before periods stop and usually are present for less than 5 years. Some women, however, will continue to flush into their 60s and 70s. Flushes are episodes of inappropriate heat loss mediated by cutaneous vasodilation over the upper trunk. Some women also complain of psychological symptoms such as tiredness, depressed mood, loss of libido and lethargy. Cultural differences in attitudes to the menopause seem to exist: for example, menopausal complaints are fewer in Japanese than in North American women. The effect of exercise on hot flushes is conflicting with some studies showing benefit and others not. Women with a higher level of education seem to have fewer symptoms.

Investigations

FOLLICLE-STIMULATING HORMONE

FSH levels are helpful only if the diagnosis of ovarian failure is in doubt and the levels are reported in the menopausal range (greater than 30 iu/l). FSH needs to be measured in women with suspected premature ovarian failure, whether or not they have had a hysterectomy. It is best to take samples on days 3–5 of the cycle (day 1 is the first day of menstruation). Where this is not possible – such as in women with oligomenorrhoea or amenorrhoea or who have undergone hysterectomy – two samples separated by an interval of 2 weeks should be obtained.

There is no need to measure FSH in women over the age of 45 years who are having hot flushes. FSH levels vary markedly on a daily basis during the perimenopause. FSH levels are not a guide to fertility status or when the last period is likely to occur. They are also of little value in monitoring

HRT, as this gonadotrophin is controlled by inhibin as well as estradiol.

LUTEINISING HORMONE, ESTRADIOL AND PROGESTERONE

Measuring luteinising hormone, estradiol and progesterone is of no value in diagnosing ovarian failure. Estradiol levels may be of some value in checking absorption of estradiol delivered by the non-oral route but not the oral route as, with the latter, the major circulating metabolite is estrone.

THYROID FUNCTION TESTS (FREE T4 AND THYROID-STIMULATING HORMONE)

Thyroid disease affects up to 20% of women. It can cause hot flushes. Therefore, thyroid function tests should be checked in women with an inadequate symptomatic response to HRT.

CATECHOLAMINES AND 5-HYDROXYINDOLACETIC ACID

Twenty-four-hour urine levels of catecholamines and 5-hydroxyindolacetic acid are used to diagnose phaeochromocytoma and carcinoid syndrome, respectively. Both are rare cause of hot flushes.

Treatment

ESTROGEN

The most effective treatment is estrogen-based HRT. Treatment should be continued for up to 5 years and then stopped to evaluate whether they have recurred. This duration will not significantly increase the risk of breast cancer.

CLONIDINE

Clonidine is a centrally acting alpha-adrenoceptor agonist that was developed originally for the treatment of hypertension. While it has been one of the most popular alternative preparations for the treatment of vasomotor symptoms since the 1980s, the evidence for efficacy is poor in RCTs. A dose of 50–75 micrograms twice daily has limited value and effectiveness.

SELECTIVE SEROTONIN REUPTAKE INHIBITORS AND SEROTONIN AND NORADRENALINE REUPTAKE INHIBITORS

Fluoxetine, paroxetine, citalopram and venlafaxine have been found to be effective in several studies. However, most are short-lasting: only a few weeks. A 9-month, placebo-controlled study of citalopram and fluoxetine showed no benefit. Further evidence is awaited. Some early evidence suggests that SSRIs may cause bone loss. New SNRIs such as desvenlafaxine are being investigated for the management of hot flushes.

GABAPENTIN

Gabapentin is a gamma-aminobutyric acid analogue used to treat epilepsy, neurogenic pain and migraine. Limited evidence has shown efficacy for hot flush reduction compared with placebo and further work is required.

PROGESTOGENS

Progestogens such as 5 mg/day norethisterone or 40 mg/day megestrol acetate can be effective in controlling hot flushes and night sweats. However, at doses that achieve control of vasomotor symptoms, the risk of venous thromboembolism is increased.

OTHERS

The antidepressants veralipride and moclobemide have also been studied. However, they are of limited effectiveness and there are concerns about adverse effects. Beta blockers were advocated in the early 1980s but, again, the evidence is poor.

Urogenital problems

Estrogen deficiency can cause vaginal atrophy and urinary problems. Vaginal atrophy is a common menopausal problem. It affects about one-third of women even if they are taking systemic HRT. Although not life threatening, vaginal atrophy can be extremely uncomfortable and can result in dyspareunia, cessation of sexual activity, itching, burning and dryness. Urinary symptoms include frequency, urgency, nocturia, incontinence and recurrent infection. Women may suffer in silence and not seek medical help.

The lower urinary and genital tracts have a common embryological origin. Estrogen and progesterone receptors are present in the vagina, urethra, bladder and pelvic floor. Thus, postmenopausal estrogen deficiency causes atrophic changes.

ASSESSMENT

Routine examination and investigations are not normally indicated unless there has been postcoital or postmenopausal bleeding or an offensive or pruritic discharge. The patient may refuse to be examined because of pain. However, if symptoms are not improved after 6 months, it would be prudent to examine her to exclude other pathologies such as lichen sclerosis.

NONHORMONAL OPTIONS

Lubricants and vaginal moisturisers are available without prescription. While being a popular first-line option, the number of published scientific trials is limited. Lubricants usually consist of a combination of protectants and thickening agents in a water-soluble base. They are usually used as temporary measures to relieve vaginal dryness during intercourse. They therefore do not provide a long-term solution. Lubricants must be applied frequently for more continuous relief and require reapplication before sexual activity. The integrity and efficacy of condoms may be compromised by lubricants such as petroleum-based products and baby oil. This is important when condoms are used to prevent sexually transmitted infections.

Moisturisers may contain a bioadhesive polycarbophil-based polymer, which attaches to mucin and epithelial cells on the vaginal wall and retains water. Moisturisers are promoted as providing long-term relief of vaginal dryness and need to be applied less frequently.

HORMONAL OPTIONS

Estrogen-based HRT is effective in treating symptoms of vaginal atrophy in postmenopausal women. Either systemic or local estrogen is effective. If a woman chooses not to take systemic therapy, the options available are low-dose natural estrogens, such as vaginal estradiol by tablet or ring (which is changed every 3 months) or estriol by cream or pessary. Estriol can also be given orally but only in women who have had a hysterectomy because of the increased risk of endometrial cancer. With the recommended vaginal estradiol and estriol regimens, no adverse endometrial effects should be incurred and a progestogen need not be added for endometrial protection with such low-dose preparations. Vaginal estrogens can also be used with systemic estrogens. As noted earlier, women taking systemic hormone therapy may still have urogenital atrophy. Vaginal estrogens may help with recurrent urinary tract infections. Systemic estrogens, however, do not improve incontinence.

DURATION OF TREATMENT WITH TOPICAL ESTROGEN

It may take several months for the symptoms to improve with vaginal estrogens. It is essential to inform the woman of this, as otherwise she might be expecting a rapid improvement similar to the response of hot flushes to systemic estrogen. Treatment is needed in the long term, if not lifelong, as symptoms return on cessation of treatment.

Sexual problems

Sexual problems in women are common. It has been estimated that problems affect about one in two women and they become more common as women get older. Interest in sex declines in both sexes with increasing age and this change is more pronounced in women. The term female sexual dysfunction is now used and an international classification system is now employed (Table 7).

The ovaries are an important source of testosterone, which is hydroxylated to dihydrotestosterone. Testosterone also can be aromatised to estradiol. Precursor estrogen hormones, such as androstenedione and DHEA, are produced in the ovaries and the adrenals, and both possess a less potent androgenic effect than testosterone. By the time women reach their mid-40s, mean circulating levels of testosterone, androstenedione, DHEA and its sulphate (DHEA-S) are approximately 50% those of women in their 20s. Menopausal status does not affect levels of androgens in women aged 45–54 years, however, and the postmenopausal ovary seems to be a continuing site of testosterone production. Low circulating levels of androgens have been proposed to be associated with low sexual desire; however, no level of a single androgen is predictive of low sexual function in women.

ASSESSMENT

Women who complain of lack of libido may request measurement of levels of testosterone. However, this may be of little value (see above). Furthermore, more than two-thirds of circulating testosterone is bound to steroid hormone-binding globulin (SHBG) and a further third is weakly bound to albumin, which leaves around 2% of the total testosterone in the free or unbound state. As concentrations of SHBG can fluctuate, total levels of testosterone do not yield meaningful information about exposure of the tissues to androgens. A free testosterone index accurately evaluates the tissue androgen status but is not available routinely in clinical practice. It is more important to take a detailed sexual history as the underlying reasons for sexual dysfunction are commonly multifactorial and male problems such as erectile difficulties should not be overlooked.

Management plans

Management plans can be divided into non-hormonal and hormonal.

NON-HORMONAL

Self-help sexual materials of all kinds are easy to find: books, DVDs, vibrators, clitoral stimulators, erotic games and lingerie. These can be easily found on the internet.

Psychosexual therapy (also referred to as sex therapy or psychosexual counselling) has proven success rates. Both partners should be encouraged

Table 7   Consensus classification system for female sexual dysfunction (adapted from Basson, 2000)

	Classification	Definition
I	**Sexual desire disorders**	
A	Hypoactive sexual desire disorder	The persistent or recurrent deficiency (or absence) of sexual fantasies/thoughts and/or desire for or receptivity to sexual activity, which causes personal distress
B	Sexual aversion disorder	The persistent or recurrent phobic aversion and avoidance of sexual contact with a sexual partner, which causes personal distress
II	**Sexual arousal disorders**	The persistent or recurrent inability to attain or maintain sufficient sexual excitement, causing personal distress, which may be expressed as a lack of subjective excitement or genital (lubrication/swelling) or other somatic responses
III	**Orgasmic disorder**	The persistent or recurrent difficulty, delay in or absence of attaining orgasm after sufficient sexual stimulation and arousal, which causes personal distress
IV	**Sexual pain disorders**	
A	Dyspareunia	The recurrent or persistent genital pain associated with sexual intercourse
B	Vaginismus	The recurrent or persistent involuntary spasm of the musculature of the outer third of the vagina, which interferes with vaginal penetration and causes personal distress
C	Noncoital sexual pain disorders	Recurrent or persistent genital pain induced by noncoital sexual stimulation

Each of the categories above is subtyped on the basis of the medical history, physical examination and laboratory tests as: (A) lifelong versus acquired; (B) generalised versus situational or (C) aetiology (organic, psychogenic, mixed or unknown).

to attend. Following initial assessment, the therapist will give the couple information about how sexual problems arise and the various treatment options available. It is important to ensure that the sex therapist is qualified and abides by the code of ethics of an appropriate professional body.

If lubrication is a problem, this may be improved by lubricants and bio-adhesive moisturisers (see above).

HORMONAL

Estrogens
Topical and systemic estrogen use is detailed above.

Testosterone
Several studies have shown a benefit of testosterone therapy in postmenopausal women but mainly in those using estrogen. In the UK, the only licensed preparations for women for many years were subcutaneous implants or pellets to be put under the skin using local anaesthesia. Testosterone patches for women are now available. These have the advantage that women can start and stop treatment whenever they want.

Tibolone
This is a synthetic steroid with similar effects to the female hormones estrogen and progesterone, as well as testosterone. It can improve menopausal symptoms such as hot flushes and can improve lack of libido.

Further reading

VASOMOTOR SYMPTOMS

Aiello EJ, Yasui Y, Tworoger SS, Ulrich CM, Irwin ML, Bowen D, et al. Effect of a yearlong, moderate-intensity exercise intervention on the occurrence and severity of menopause symptoms in postmenopausal women. *Menopause* 2004;11:382–8.

Deecher DC, Alfinito PD, Leventhal L, Cosmi S, Johnston GH, Merchenthaler I, et al. Alleviation of thermoregulatory dysfunction with the new serotonin and norepinephrine reuptake inhibitor desvenlafaxine succinate in ovariectomized rodent models. *Endocrinology* 2007;148:1376–83.

Diem SJ, Blackwell TL, Stone KL, Yaffe K, Haney EM, Bliziotes MM, Ensrud KE. Use of antidepressants and rates of hip bone loss in older women: the study of osteoporotic fractures. *Arch Intern Med* 2007;167:1240–5.

Lindh-Astrand L, Nedstrand E, Wyon Y, Hammar M.Vasomotor symptoms and quality of life in previously sedentary postmenopausal women randomised to physical activity or estrogen therapy. *Maturitas* 2004;48:97–105.

Lock M. Symptom reporting at menopause: a review of cross-cultural findings. *J Br Menopause Soc* 2002;8:132–6.

Loprinzi CL, Michalak JC, Quella SK, O'Fallon JR, Hatfield AK, Nelimark RA, *et al.* Megestrol acetate for the prevention of hot flashes. *N Eng J Med* 1994; 331:347–52.

Nelson HD, Vesco KK, Haney E, Fu R, Nedrow A, Miller J, *et al.* Nonhormonal therapies for menopausal hot flashes: systematic review and meta-analysis. *JAMA* 2006;295:2057–71.

Nedrow A, Miller J, Walker M, Nygren P, Huffman LH, Nelson HD. Complementary and alternative therapies for the management of menopause-related symptoms: a systematic evidence review. *Arch Intern Med* 2006;166:1453–65.

Rees M, Purdie DW. *Management of the Menopause. The Handbook.* 4th ed. London: Royal Society of Medicine Press; 2006.

Suvanto-Luukkonen E, Koivunen R, Sundström H, Bloigu R, Karjalainen E, Häivä-Mällinen L, *et al.* Citalopram and fluoxetine in the treatment of postmenopausal symptoms: a prospective, randomized, 9-month, placebo-controlled, double-blind study. *Menopause* 2005;12:18–26.

Thurston RC, Joffe H, Soares CN, Harlow BL. Physical activity and risk of vasomotor symptoms in women with and without a history of depression: results from the Harvard Study of Moods and Cycles. *Menopause* 2006;13: 553–60.

Vasilakis C, Jick H, del Mar Melero-Montes M. Risk of idiopathic venous thromboembolism in users of progestagens alone. *Lancet* 1999;354:1610–11.

Whitcomb BW, Whiteman MK, Langenberg P, Flaws JA, Romani WA. Physical activity and risk of hot flashes among women in midlife. *J Womens Health (Larchmt)* 2007;16:124–33.

UROGENITAL PROBLEMS

Bygdeman M, Swahn ML. Replens versus dienoestrol cream in the symptomatic treatment of vaginal atrophy in postmenopausal women. *Maturitas* 1996;23:259–63.

Castelo-Branco C, Cancelo MJ, Villero J, Nohales F, Julia MD. Management of post-menopausal vaginal atrophy and atrophic vaginitis. *Maturitas* 2005;52(Suppl 1):S46–52.

Franco AV. Recurrent urinary tract infections. *Best Pract Res Clin Obstet Gynaecol* 2005;19:861–73.

Hendrix SL, Cochrane BB, Nygaard IE, Handa VL, Barnabei VM, Iglesia C, *et al.* Effects of estrogen with and without progestin on urinary incontinence. *JAMA* 2005;293:935–48.

Oskay UY, Beji NK, Yalcin O. A study on urogenital complaints of postmenopausal women aged 50 and over. *Acta Obstet Gynecol Scand* 2005;84:72–8.

Rosen AD, Rosen T. Study of condom integrity after brief exposure to over-the-counter vaginal preparations. *South Med J* 1999;92:305–7.

Simunić V, Banović I, Ciglar S, Jeren L, Pavicić Baldani D, Sprem M. Local estrogen treatment in patients with urogenital symptoms. *Int J Gynaecol Obstet* 2003;82:187–97.

Suckling J, Lethaby A, Kennedy R. Local oestrogen for vaginal atrophy in postmenopausal women. *Cochrane Database Syst Rev* 2006;(4):CD001500.

Weisberg E, Ayton R, Darling G, Farrell E, Murkies A, O'Neill S, *et al.* Endometrial and vaginal effects of low-dose estradiol delivered by vaginal ring or vaginal tablet. *Climacteric* 2005;8:83–92.

SEXUAL PROBLEMS

Basson R, Berman J, Burnett A, Derogatis L, Ferguson D, Fourcroy J, *et al.* Report of the international consensus development conference on female sexual dysfunction: definitions and classifications. *J Urol* 2000;163:888–93.

Davis SR, Davison SL, Donath S, Bell RJ. Circulating androgen levels and self-reported sexual function in women. *JAMA* 2005;294:91–6.

Davis SR, van der Mooren MJ, van Lunsen RH, Lopes P, Ribot C, Rees M, *et al.* Efficacy and safety of a testosterone patch for the treatment of hypoactive sexual desire disorder in surgically menopausal women: a randomized, placebo-controlled trial. *Menopause* 2006;13:387–96 [Erratum in: *Menopause* 2006;13(5):850. Ribot, Jean corrected to Ribot, Claude].

Dennerstein L, Alexander JL, Kotz K. The menopause and sexual functioning: a review of the population-based studies. *Annu Rev Sex Res* 2003;14:64–82.

Egarter C, Topcuoglu A, Vogl S, Sator M. Hormone replacement therapy with tibolone: effects on sexual functioning in postmenopausal women. *Acta Obstet Gynecol Scand* 2002;81:649–53.

Kingsberg S. Testosterone treatment for hypoactive sexual desire disorder in postmenopausal women. *J Sex Med* 2007;4(Suppl 3):227–34.

Lindau ST, Schumm LP, Laumann EO, Levinson W, O'Muircheartaigh CA, Waite LJ. A study of sexuality and health among older adults in the United States. *N Engl J Med* 2007;357:762–74.

Sexual Dysfunction Association [www.sda.uk.net].

Tomlinson JM, Rees M, Mander T, editors. *Sexual Health and the Menopause.* London: RSM Press and British Menopause Society Publications; 2005.

8 Osteoporosis and autoimmune arthritis

Osteoporosis

Osteoporosis is a major problem with one in three women over 50 years and one in 12 men having one or more osteoporotic fracture. The lifetime risk (percent) in the USA for a hip, spine or forearm fracture at the age of 50 years has been estimated to be 40% in women and 13% in men.

DEFINITION

Osteoporosisis is defined in a US National Institutes of Health consensus statement as 'a skeletal disorder characterised by compromised bone strength predisposing to an increased risk of fracture'. Bone strength reflects the integration of two main features: bone density and bone quality. Bone density is expressed as grams of mineral per area or volume and, in any given individual, is determined by peak bone mass and amount of bone loss. Bone quality refers to architecture, turnover, damage accumulation (for example, microfractures) and mineralisation.

On the basis of the measurement of bone mineral density (BMD), the World Health Organization's definitions (Box 4), result in 30% of post-menopausal women being classified as having osteoporosis. The 'T' score is

---

BOX 4. DEFINITIONS OF OSTEOPOROSIS ACCORDING TO THE WORLD HEALTH ORGANIZATION

Normal   A person has a BMD value between −1 SD and +1 SD of the young adult mean (T score −1 to +1)

Osteopenia   A person has a BMD reduced between −1 and −2.5 SD from the young adult mean (T score −1 to −2.5)

Osteoporosis A person has a BMD reduced by equal to or more than −2.5 SD from the young adult mean
(T score −2.5 or lower)

---

that number of standard deviations (SD) by which a particular bone differs from the young normal mean.

OSTEOPOROTIC FRACTURES

Fractures are the clinical consequences of osteoporosis. The most common sites of osteoporotic fractures are the wrist (or Colles' fracture), the hip and the spine. Other sites include the pelvis, ribs, humerus and distal femur. The cost of osteoporotic fracture is high. For example, the cost for hip fractures worldwide is estimated to be US$34,800 million in 1990 and to reach US$131,500 million in 2050. Fractures have a major impact on quality of life, result in a significant economic burden and, particularly in the case of hip fractures, are associated with considerable excess mortality. In the year after a hip fracture, mortality is about 30%. About 50% of patients who survive hip fracture have permanent disability and fail to regain their previous level of independence.

DETERMINANTS OF BONE MASS

Age

Bone density increases in the teenage years, reaching a peak during the mid-20s. Peak bone density is then sustained for some years and begins to decline during the mid-40s. After the menopause, an accelerated phase of bone loss occurs, which lasts for 6–10 years. Thereafter, bone loss continues but at a much slower rate (Figure 1). Any bone has a 'threshold'

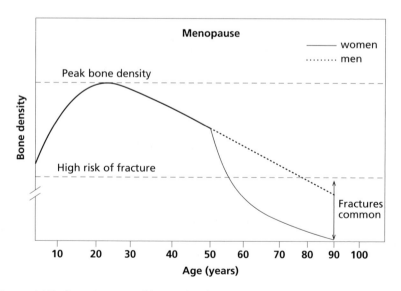

Figure 1 Lifetime changes of bone density

value of bone mass below which the bone will fracture after minor trauma. Although low bone mass is a major contributor to risk of fracture, other factors, including age, body mass index, falls and bone quality, contribute to whether a person will sustain a fracture.

Sex

Whether a postmenopausal woman develops osteoporosis is determined by her peak bone mass, rate of postmenopausal bone loss and her age. Men have fewer osteoporotic fractures than women because they have a much higher peak bone mass and do not have the postmenopausal accelerated phase of bone loss.

Ethnic group

There are ethnic variations in the susceptibility to osteoporosis. For example white women have a higher rate of fracture than those of African-Caribbean origin.

Genetic phenotypes such as BMD, femoral neck geometry, quantitative ultrasound properties of bone and biochemical markers of bone turnover are largely under genetic control. Twin studies and family-based studies have indicated that as much as 60–85% of the variance in BMD is

---

BOX 5. RISK FACTORS FOR OSTEOPOROSIS

Genetic	Family history of fracture (particularly a first-degree relative with hip fracture)
Constitutional	Low body mass index Early menopause (less than 45 years of age)
Environmental	Cigarette smoking Alcohol abuse Low calcium intake Sedentary life style
Drugs	Corticosteroids, greater than 5 mg prednisolone or equivalent daily
Diseases	Rheumatoid arthritis Neuromuscular disease Chronic liver disease Malabsorption syndromes Hyperparathyroidism Hyperthyroidism Hypogonadism

genetically determined and heritability estimates for other risk factors for fragility fracture, such as quantitative ultrasound, femoral neck geometry and bone turnover markers, range between 50% and 80%. A family history of fracture is a significant risk factor for fracture but the heritability of fracture itself is relatively low (25–35%), reflecting the importance of fall-related factors in the pathogenesis of fracture.

It is unlikely that a single gene defect exists for osteoporosis but several candidates that influence BMD have been examined, including those for the vitamin D receptor, estrogen receptor, collagen type 1, transforming growth factor beta-1 and lipoprotein receptor-related protein-5.

RISK FACTORS FOR THE DEVELOPMENT OF OSTEOPOROSIS

Risk factors for osteoporotic fracture are detailed in Box 5. The factors most important in clinical practice are parental history of fracture (particularly hip fracture), early menopause, chronic use of corticosteroids (oral and possibly inhaled), prolonged immobilisation and prior fracture.

Depot medroxyprogesterone acetate (DMPA) provides an effective form of contraception. However, there are concerns about the induced bone loss. While bone loss occurs early on during treatment, it is not progressive and reverses on ceasing DMPA. It is probably prudent to discontinue DMPA at the age of 40 years to allow resumption of ovarian cycling for the remaining 10 years or so up to the natural menopause. The long-term skeletal effects of DMPA in teenagers who have yet to achieve peak bone mass are uncertain and have to be balanced against the benefits of an effective form of contraception. It would also be advisable to assess an individual's risk for osteoporosis before prescribing DMPA.

INVESTIGATIONS

Bone density estimation
It is generally agreed that population screening is of little value and that it is better to target women at risk of osteoporosis (Box 5).

Dual energy X-ray absorptiometry
Dual energy X-ray absorptiometry (DXA) is an X-ray-based system that uses two different energies to differentiate between soft tissue and bone. The X-rays are directed anterior–posterior or vice versa, depending on the instrument. Fan-beam and pencil-beam machines can scan laterally around the side of a patient, which is useful for measuring the bone density of the lumbar spine.

Values for BMD may be quoted as g/cm^2 or converted into values that relate to either the average female (or male) peak bone mass (T score) or that of the patient's age group (Z score):

$$\text{T score} = \frac{\text{patient's BMD} - \text{population peak BMD}}{\text{SD of population peak BMD}}$$

$$\text{Z score} = \frac{\text{patient's BMD} - \text{population age-related BMD}}{\text{SD of population age-related BMD}}$$

Calibrations for average bone densities are often based on a US database of the upper femur, called the National Health and Nutrition Examination Survey (NHANES) database.

The main sites for measurement are the spine (L1 or L2–L4) and various regions of interest at the hip. Since the spine may have falsely increased values due to osteophytes from osteoarthritis, kyphosis, scoliosis and aortic calcification, it now is recommended that the best site to measure is the hip. BMD of the 'total hip' and the neck of femur are the most commonly used measurements. Peripheral DXA (pDXA) systems measure the forearm or calcaneus and may be considered to be a risk assessment tool. They cannot, however, replace hip DXA for the formal diagnosis of osteoporosis.

The frequency of follow-up scans is controversial. Initially, follow-up scans may be undertaken at 2 years to assess response to treatment and, in general, should not be performed more frequently than every 3 years thereafter. In the USA, most private healthcare plans provide coverage for BMD testing to monitor the therapeutic response to therapy but they will not generally reimburse testing for this indication more often than every 2 years.

Single-energy X-ray absorptiometry
This method is used commonly for wrist scans.

Quantitative computed tomography
Quantitative computed tomography provides measurement of the spine, hip and wrist. It does not have a diagnostic ability superior to that of DXA. Its use in clinical practice is limited by poorer precision and much higher radiation doses than used with DXA.

Quantitative ultrasound
This technique involves the transmission of a low-amplitude ultrasound beam, usually through the calcaneus, which measures bone strength. It does not use ionising radiation and the devices are portable. It remains to be evaluated fully before it can be used in routine clinical practice. In terms of diagnostic capability, most data involve prediction of fractures in elderly women, where it is able to assess the risk of hip fracture. However, it is

uncertain whether it can predict fracture at other sites or in younger menopausal women.

Biochemical markers of bone metabolism

Biochemical markers of bone turnover are classified as markers of resorption or formation (Box 6). Most markers of bone resorption are products of collagen degradation that are released into the circulation and finally excreted in the urine. Tartrate-resistant acid phosphatase is secreted by osteoclasts and levels are measured in serum. Markers of bone formation are by-products of collagen formation, matrix proteins or enzymes associated with osteoblast activity.

Since bone resorption and formation are 'coupled' processes in most situations, any marker can be used to determine the overall rate of bone turnover. Biochemical markers of bone turnover are particularly attractive as a means of monitoring therapeutic efficacy because significant suppression of bone turnover occurs far more rapidly than detectable changes in bone mineral density. They reach a nadir within 3–6 months of initiation of therapy in clinical trials. However, the imprecision of

---

BOX 6. MOST COMMONLY USED BIOCHEMICAL MARKERS OF BONE TURNOVER (adapted from Hannon, 2003)

Bone formation

By-products of collagen synthesis:
- pro-collagen type 1 C terminal pro-peptide (PICP)[a]
- pro-collagen type 1 N terminal pro-peptide (PINP)[a]

Matrix protein:
- osteocalcin (OC)[a]

Osteoblast enzyme:
- total alkaline phosphatase (total ALP)[a]
- bone alkaline phosphatase (bone ALP)[a]

Bone resorption

Collagen degradation products:
- hydroxyproline (Hyp)[b]
- pyridinoline (PYD)[a,b]
- deoxypyridinoline (DPD)[a,b]

Crosslinked telopeptides of type I collagen:
- N-terminal crosslinked telopeptide (NTX)[a,b]
- C-terminal crosslinked telopeptide (CTX)[a,b]
- C-terminal crosslinked telopeptide generated by matrix metalloproteinases (MMPs) (CTX-MMP, formerly ICTP)[a]

Osteoclast enzyme:
- Tartrate-resistant acid phosphatase (TRACP)[a]
- osteocalcin (OC)[a]

a = measured in serum   b = measured in urine

---

measuring bone turnover using markers is far greater than that of measuring bone mineral density using DXA and cutoff values for the use of markers of bone turnover are uncertain.

TREATMENT OF OSTEOPOROSIS

Specific treatments have already been described in Chapters 3, 4 and 5. There is evidence from RCTs, including the WHI, that HRT reduces the risk of both spine and hip as well as other osteoporotic fractures. The standard bone-conserving doses of estrogen were considered to be estradiol 2 mg, conjugated equine estrogens 0.625 mg and transdermal 50-microgram patch. However, it is now evident that lower doses also conserve bone mass. Most epidemiological studies suggest that for HRT to be an effective method of preventing fracture, continuous and lifelong use is required. However, it has now been shown that just a few years of treatment with HRT around the time of menopause may have a long-term effect on fracture reduction. Regulatory authorities (December 2003) have advised that HRT should not be used as a first-line treatment for osteoporosis prevention as the risks outweigh the benefits. This may be true for a population with no increased osteoporosis risk, as in WHI, but the risk–benefit ratio changes favourably when targeting a population with increased osteoporosis risk. While alternatives to HRT use are available for the prevention and treatment of osteoporosis in elderly women, estrogen may still remain the best option, particularly in younger (less than 60 years) and/or symptomatic women. Estrogen remains the treatment of choice in women with premature ovarian failure. No clinical trial evidence attests the efficacy or safety of the use of non-estrogen-based treatments, such as bisphosphonates, strontium ranelate or raloxifene, in these women. The initiation of 'standard dose' HRT is not recommended solely for fracture prevention in women over 60 years of age.

Although some women will be happy to take HRT for life, others may view treatment as a continuum of options and will wish to change to other agents such as a bisphosphonate or strontium ranelate, because of the small but measurable increase in risk of breast cancer associated with the long-term use of combined HRT.

Hip protectors are used to reduce the impact of falling directly on the hip but evidence of efficacy is conflicting. Systematic review has found no evidence of effectiveness of hip protectors from studies in which randomisation was by individual patient within an institution or for those living in their own homes. Data from randomised cluster studies indicate that, for those who live in institutional care with a high background incidence of hip fracture, a programme in which hip protectors are provided seems to reduce the incidence of hip fractures. However, a randomised study of nursing home residents showed no benefit. An RCT of women older than 70 years at high risk of hip fracture who lived in the community in the UK found no benefit.

Autoimmune disease

RHEUMATOID ARTHRITIS

Rheumatoid arthritis is a chronic, systemic, inflammatory autoimmune disease that has as its primary target the synovial tissues. When the disease is unchecked, it leads to substantial disability and premature death. It affects approximately 0.8% of adults worldwide, is more common in women (by a ratio of three to one) and has an earlier onset in women, frequently beginning in the childbearing years. Women with rheumatoid arthritis are at increased risk of osteoporosis and this may be related to disease severity, steroid use and immobility caused by the disease. Furthermore, bone resorption is increased in women with rheumatoid arthritis and this is related to disease activity. The use of estrogen or non-estrogen-based treatments will depend on the woman's symptoms, bone mineral density and preference. No evidence shows that the use of HRT affects the risk of developing rheumatoid arthritis and it does not induce flares in menopausal women. It may reduce inflammation and slow progression of radiological joint destruction. Bisphosphonates also are effective at reducing fracture.

SYSTEMIC LUPUS ERYTHMATOSUS

Systemic lupus erythematosus (SLE) is a multi-system rheumatic disease characterised by fever, arthritis, pleuropericarditis, skin rashes, grand mal seizures, kidney failure or pancytopenia. It has a female male ratio of nine to one between puberty and the menopause. Classically, it is considered that estrogen may worsen the course of the disease, in particular, pregnancy and oral contraceptives. Recent randomised trials, however, have shown that oral contraceptives may not be as deleterious as previously thought. It is usually considered that SLE is a contraindication to HRT because of the hormone-dependency of the disease. However, women with SLE are susceptible to premature ovarian failure from autoimmune disease or cyclophosphamide treatment and thus menopause seems to occur at a younger age. The increased life expectancy of patients with SLE means that early cardiovascular mortality and glucocorticoid-associated bone loss are now important issues. Surveys have found that fractures occur in 12.3% of patients with SLE. The occurrence of fracture in women with SLE is now five-fold higher than that in normal women. Older age at diagnosis of SLE and longer use of corticosteroids are associated with time from diagnosis of SLE to fracture.

HRT can induce SLE flares and cardiovascular or venous thrombo-embolic events. Thus, it should not be used in women with active disease or those with antiphospholipid (aPL) antibodies. In general it should only be used in patients without active disease, history of thrombosis or aPL antibodies. Non-oral estrogen administration is recommended because of its lesser effect on coagulation. With regard to the progestogen, progesterone or pregnane derivatives are preferred.

With regard to osteoporosis, bisphosphonates have been studied in glucocorticoid induced osteoporosis and can be used in conjunction with calcium and vitamin D and exercise. Strontium ranelate mildly increases venous thromboembolic risk and is thus probably best avoided. While raloxifene conserves bone mass in women with SLE, it is probably also best avoided in those at risk of venous thromboembolism.

Lifestyle interventions can also be employed as in other menopausal women. Maintaining a normal BMI, exercising, stopping smoking and maintaining an adequate intake of calcium and vitamin D are all advisable.

Further reading

OSTEOPOROSIS

Bagger YZ, Tankó LB, Alexandersen P, Hansen HB, Møllgaard A, Ravn P, *et al.* Two to three years of hormone replacement treatment in healthy women have long-term preventive effects on bone mass and osteoporotic fractures: the PERF study. *Bone* 2004;34:728–35.

Bonnick SL, Shulman L. Monitoring osteoporosis therapy: bone mineral density, bone turnover markers, or both? *Am J Med* 2006;119(4 Suppl 1): S25–31.

Cauley JA, Robbins J, Chen Z, Cummings SR, Jackson RD, LaCroix AZ, *et al;* Women's Health Initiative Investigators. Effects of estrogen plus progestin on risk of fracture and bone mineral density: the Women's Health Initiative randomized trial. *JAMA* 2003;290:1729–38.

Clark MK, Sowers M, Levy B, Nichols S. Bone mineral density loss and recovery during 48 months in first-time users of depot medroxyprogesterone acetate. *Fertil Steril* 2006;86:1466–74.

Committee on Safety of Medicines. Further advice on safety of HRT: risk : benefit unfavourable for first-line use in prevention of osteoporosis. CEM/CMO/2003/19 [www.mhra.gov.uk/home/idcplg?IdcService=GET_FILE &dDocName=con019496&RevisionSelectionMethod=Latest].

Ettinger B, Ensrud KE, Wallace R, Johnson KC, Cummings SR, Yankov V, *et al.* Effects of ultralow-dose transdermal estradiol on bone mineral density: a randomized clinical trial. *Obstet Gynecol* 2004;104:443–51.

Hannon RA, Eastell R. Biochemical markers of bone turnover and fracture prediction. *J Br Menopause Soc* 2003;9:10–15.

Johnell O. The socioeconomic burden of fractures: today and in the 21st century. *Am J Med* 1997;103:20–5S.

Johnell O, Kanis J. Epidemiology of osteoporotic fractures. *Osteoporos Int* 2005;16(Suppl 2):S3–7.

Kiel DP, Magaziner J, Zimmerman S, Ball L, Barton BA, Brown KM, Stone JP, Dewkett D, Birge SJ. Efficacy of a hip protector to prevent hip fracture in nursing home residents: the HIP PRO randomized controlled trial. *JAMA* 2007;298:413–22.

National Institutes of Health, Consensus Development Panel on Osteoporosis Prevention, Diagnosis, and Therapy. Osteoporosis prevention, diagnosis, and therapy. *JAMA* 2001;285:785–95.

Poole KES, Compston JE. Osteoporosis and its management. *BMJ* 2006;333:1251–6.

Ralston SH. Genetic determinants of osteoporosis. *Curr Opin Rheumatol* 2005;17:475–9.

Scholes D, LaCroix AZ, Ichikawa LE, Barlow WE, Ott SM. Change in bone mineral density among adolescent women using and discontinuing depot medroxyprogesterone acetate contraception. *Arch Pediatr Adolesc Med* 2005;159:139–44.

Stevenson JC; International Consensus Group on HRT and Regulatory Issues. HRT, osteoporosis and regulatory authorities: Quis custodiet ipsos custodes? *Hum Reprod* 2006;21:1668–71.

Women's Health Initiative Steering Committee. Effects of conjugated equine estrogen in postmenopausal women with hysterectomy: the Women's Health Initiative randomized controlled trial. *JAMA* 2004;291:1701–12.

World Health Organization. Assessment of fracture risk and its application to screening for postmenopausal osteoporosis. Report of a WHO Study Group. *WHO Tech Rep Ser* 1994;843:1–129.

Writing Group on Osteoporosis for the British Menopause Society Council, Al-Azzawi F, Barlow D, Hillard T, Studd J, Williamson J, Rees M. Prevention and treatment of ostroporosis in women. *Menopause Int* 2007;13:178–81.

AUTOIMMUNE ARTHRITIS

Canonico M, Oger E, Plu-Bureau G, Conard J, Meyer G, Lévesque H, et al; Estrogen and Thromboembolism Risk (ESTHER) Study Group. Hormone therapy and venous thromboembolism among postmenopausal women: impact of the route of estrogen administration and progestogens: the ESTHER study. *Circulation* 2007;115:840–5.

D'Elia HF, Larsen A, Mattsson LA, Waltbrand E, Kvist G, Mellström D, et al. Influence of hormone replacement therapy on disease progression and bone mineral density in rheumatoid arthritis. *J Rheumatol* 2003;30:1456–63.

Gompel A, Piette JC. Systemic lupus erythematosus and hormone replacement therapy. *Menopause Int* 2007;13:65–70.

Hall GM, Daniels M, Huskisson EC, Spector TD. A randomised controlled trial of the effect of hormone replacement therapy on disease activity in postmenopausal rheumatoid arthritis. *Ann Rheum Dis* 1994;53:112–16.

Koepsell TD, Dugowson CE, Nelson JL, Voigt LF, Daling JR. Non-contraceptive hormones and the risk of rheumatoid arthritis in menopausal women. *Int J Epidemiol* 1994;23:1248–55.

Lange U, Illgner U, Teichmann J, Schleenbecker H. Skeletal benefit after one year of risedronate therapy in patients with rheumatoid arthritis and glucocorticoid-induced osteoporosis: a prospective study. *Int J Clin Pharmacol Res* 2004;24:33–8.

Lodder MC, de Jong Z, Kostense PJ, Molenaar ET, Staal K, Voskuyl AE, *et al.* Bone mineral density in patients with rheumatoid arthritis: relation between disease severity and low bone mineral density. *Ann Rheum Dis* 2004;63:1576–80.

Mok CC, To CH, Mak A, Ma KM. Raloxifene for postmenopausal women with systemic lupus erythematosus: a pilot randomized controlled study. *Arthritis Rheum* 2005;52:3997–4002.

O'Dell JR. Therapeutic strategies for rheumatoid arthritis. *N Engl J Med* 2004;17;350:2591–602.

O'Donnell S, Cranney A, Wells GA, Adachi JD, Reginster JY. Strontium ranelate for preventing and treating postmenopausal osteoporosis. *Cochrane Database Syst Rev* 2006;18;(4):CD005326.

Orcel P. Prevention and treatment of glucocorticoid-induced osteoporosis in 2005. *Joint Bone Spine* 2005;72:461–5.

Phillips K, Aliprantis A, Coblyn J. Strategies for the prevention and treatment of osteoporosis in patients with rheumatoid arthritis. *Drugs Aging* 2006;23:773–9.

9   Breast disease

Breast cancer

Worldwide, more than a million women are diagnosed with breast cancer every year, accounting for 10% of all new cancers and 23% of all female cancer cases. Breast cancer incidence rates vary considerably, with the highest rates in the developed world and the lowest rates in Africa and Asia. The lifetime risk (to 85 years of age) of developing breast cancer in developed countries worldwide is 11% (one in nine). Around 361 000 new cases of breast cancer occur each year in Europe and 210 000 in the USA. The lowest European rates are in eastern and southern Europe and the highest are in Denmark, Belgium, Sweden and the Netherlands.

Virtually all invasive breast cancers are adenocarcinomas (derived from glandular tissue), either ductal (85%) or lobular (15%). Some breast cancers are called *in situ* since they have not yet spread beyond the area where they began. The presence of lobular carcinoma *in situ* increases the risk of developing cancer in either breast, whereas ductal carcinoma *in situ* (DCIS) may progress to invasive cancer within the affected breast. DCIS is now detected more frequently because of the widespread use of mammography.

RISK FACTORS FOR BREAST CANCER

Several factors are associated with an increased risk of breast cancer (age, family history, age at first full-term pregnancy, early menarche and late menopause) (Table 8). The strongest risk factors for breast cancer are age and family history, especially a first-degree relative (see below). Some risk factors increase lifetime exposure to estrogen (early menarche, late menopause, obesity, use of HRT).

Overall, HRT seems to confer a similar degree of risk to that associated with late natural menopause. The risk of breast cancer increases by 2.8% for every year that the menopause is delayed. With HRT, the risk has been estimated to increase by 2.3% per year. Epidemiological and randomised studies suggest that the risk of developing breast cancer with HRT depends on the duration of treatment and falls when HRT is stopped. Thus, the risk after 5 years is no greater than that in women who have never taken HRT. All risk estimates are based in women starting HRT at 50 years and such an effect is not seen in those with a premature menopause.

Table 8   Breast cancer risk (adapted from American Cancer Society, 2007)

Level of increased risk (relative risk)	Risk factor
High (> 4)	Certain inherited genetic mutations, e.g. *BRCA1* or *BRCA2* Personal history breast cancer Age (65+ versus < 65 years)
Moderate (2.1–4.0)	Biopsy-confirmed atypical hyperplasia High-dose radiation to chest (mantle radiotherapy for Hodgkin's at age < 35 years)
Low (1.1–2.0)	Recent and long-term use of HRT Late age at first full term pregnancy (> 30 years) Early menarche (< 12 years) Late menopause (> 55 years) Nulliparity Alcohol consumption Postmenopausal obesity Height (tall) High socioeconomic status

The risk of breast cancer with HRT depends on the regimen. Risk seems to be greatest with combined estrogen–progestogen replacement and less so with unopposed estrogen (see Chapter 1). The estrogen-alone arm of the WHI found no increased risk of breast cancer.

Combined HRT probably accounts for an extra three breast cancers per 1000 women who start it at the age of 50 years and use it for 5 years. The increased risk of breast cancer with combined therapy compared with estrogen alone treatment has to be balanced against the reduction in risk of endometrial cancer provided by progestogen addition. The increased risk of breast cancer with longer-term exposure seems to be limited in most studies to lean women (that is those with a BMI less than 25 kg/m^2). The effect of testosterone on breast cancer risk is uncertain.

Mortality from breast cancer is the most important outcome. It is unlikely that any randomised trial, including WHI, will be large enough to evaluate this endpoint reliably. Overall, observational studies suggest that use of HRT has no significant effect on survival and may improve it. The Million Women Study reported an increased mortality in current users of HRT but this was of borderline significance. The WHI study reported that cancers associated with combined HRT were significantly larger and more likely to be node-positive than cancers associated with placebo. However, the mean difference in tumour size was only 2 mm. On the basis of data from the WHI study, the estimated survival difference at 10 years is very small (1.5%).

PREVIOUS BREAST CANCER AND HRT

Survival rates are increasing and it has been estimated that about 172000 women are alive in the UK having had a diagnosis of breast cancer. The reduction in breast cancer mortality rates is likely to have several different causes including screening, increasing specialisation of care and the widespread use of tamoxifen since the early 1990s.

Breast cancer survivors with menopausal symptoms pose a management problem, as traditional advice is to avoid the use of exogenous estrogens. They are also at increased risk of osteoporotic fracture as a result of their anticancer chemotherapy, which induces ovarian failure, gonadotrophin-releasing hormone (GnRH) analogues or aromatase inhibitors. Observational and retrospective studies in breast cancer survivors have not shown an increased risk of tumour recurrence or increased mortality associated with systemic HRT use. However, these involved small numbers of patients, with short-term follow-up, and are different in terms of lymph node status, estrogen receptor status and type of HRT used.

Early interim analysis of two randomised trials in Scandinavia (HABITS and Stockholm studies) have shown contradictory results. The increased risk of recurrence reported in HABITS has been suggested to be explained by the fact that most women randomised to HRT did not use concurrent tamoxifen and most used continuous combined HRT, whereas, in the Stockholm study, most women took tamoxifen and had long-cycle combined HRT. The adverse results of the HABITS study, although based on a very small number of clinical events, resulted in the premature cessation of the Stockholm study (in which no increase in risk was found). Currently, the effect of HRT is uncertain. The randomised LIBERATE trial of tibolone in survivors of breast cancer was stopped in July 2007 before its planned completion date.

Low-dose vaginal estrogens are not contraindicated for women with vaginal symptoms (see Chapter 7). Women with breast cancer who have severe menopausal symptoms or in whom concerns exist about osteoporosis require guidance from oncologists or menopause specialists.

Familial breast cancer

It is estimated that 5–10% of breast cancer cases result from inherited mutations or alterations in the breast cancer susceptibility genes *BRCA1*, *BRCA2*, *TP53* and *PTEN*. These mutations are present in less than 1% of the general population. However, women with Jewish ancestry are around 5–10 times more likely to carry *BRCA1* or *BRCA2* mutations than women in non-Jewish populations. Women with mutations in either *BRCA1* or *BRCA2* have a predicted lifetime risk of breast cancer between 37–85% and also of ovarian cancer between 15–40%. Other breast cancer susceptibility genes are likely to be identified. Breast cancer genes can be inherited through both sexes; family members may transmit these genes without developing cancer themselves (penetrance is variable).

Current options for patients who have been identified as being at high risk of breast cancer include prophylactic surgery, increased surveillance (see below) and chemoprevention. Several studies have shown that prophylactic mastectomy reduces the risk of breast cancer in women at high risk and specifically in *BRCA* mutation carriers. Prophylactic mastectomy is an irreversible decision and the woman should receive detailed counselling. Although mastectomy significantly reduces breast cancer mortality, it does not completely reduce the risk of breast cancer, as some breast tissue may be left behind. Nonetheless, prophylactic mastectomy with or without immediate reconstruction may be the best risk reduction option for some women at high risk.

A second primary prevention option for women is prophylactic oophorectomy. Although often considered as a risk reduction intervention for ovarian cancer, prophylactic oophorectomy has been shown to reduce the risk of breast cancer in premenopausal women and women with hereditary breast and ovarian cancer. A 50% reduction in breast cancer among *BRCA1/2* mutation carriers has been reported. These women are also at risk for ovarian cancer and oophorectomy has been shown to decrease the risk of ovarian cancer by 85–96%. Since screening for ovarian cancer has limitations, prophylactic oophorectomy may be recommended for *BRCA1/2* mutation carriers at the age of 35 years or after completion of childbearing. One concern with prophylactic oophorectomy is the induction of a premature menopause (see Chapter 11). However, HRT, especially with estrogen alone, does not increase breast cancer risk significantly in *BRCA1/2* mutation carriers.

Tamoxifen, raloxifene and aromatase inhibitors may be considered in the chemoprevention of breast cancer in women at high risk and have been studied in clinical trials. However, there are currently no available agents for the prevention of estrogen receptor-negative breast cancer.

Screening for breast cancer

MAMMOGRAPHY

Use of mammography and screening programmes varies throughout the world. No evidence supports routine mammography in women about to start HRT and no evidence suggests that women taking HRT require mammography more frequently. In the UK, the NHSBSP offers mammograms every 3 years to women aged 50–70 years. Screening is also available for older women but there is no automatic invitation. Observational studies show that HRT increases breast density on mammography. However, randomised placebo-controlled trials (including WHI and Progestin Estrogen–Progestin Intervention (PEPI) studies), have shown that not all HRT regimens have this effect. Unopposed estrogen (that is, conjugated equine estrogen) does not seem to induce any increase in density, whereas combined therapy (both cyclical and continuous combined) does, on average, in one in four women who take it. Also if any increase in density occurs, it all takes place within the first year of exposure and no evidence shows that duration of use influences this effect. The PEPI and WHI trials additionally reported that the individual degree of increase in density associated with exposure to combined HRT is in the order of 3–6%. Currently, published data from placebo-controlled randomised trials that evaluated the effect of unopposed estradiol on mammographic density and observational studies are inconsistent. At present, studies suggest that breast density on mammography is unlikely to be affected by current use of HRT in most women who participate in the UK NHSBSP.

Withdrawal of HRT before mammography has been reported to result in regression of increases in density associated with HRT sufficient to enable more accurate film reading. This question has not been subject to controlled evaluation but observational data suggest that this regression of density can occur in as little as 2 weeks. However, in the combined HRT component of the WHI study, where women who used HRT were advised to stop their therapy for 3 months before randomisation, no difference was seen in the proportion of abnormal mammograms at baseline, which supports a screening benefit for withdrawal of HRT. The MWS contrasts with placebo-controlled evidence as it reported that both unopposed and combined HRT increase density.

By increasing breast density, combined HRT can reduce the sensitivity and specificity of mammography. This would be expected to result in an increase in interval cancers (or cancers missed during screening because of decreased sensitivity) and has been reported in observational studies such as the MWS. Interval cancers diagnosed in women who take HRT have not been reported to have more adverse prognostic features, but, these data are from uncontrolled studies. Results from the randomised WHI study about interval cancers and their biological characteristics are awaited.

GENETIC TESTING

Counselling and screening must be undertaken only in specialised centres because of the ethical and legal implications. The woman's decision to undergo genetic screening is complicated by the still incomplete understanding of the penetrance of disease in known mutation carriers.

SCREENING WOMEN AT RISK OF FAMILIAL BREAST CANCER

In the UK, the National Institute for Health and Clinical Excellence has produced clinical guidance for the classification and care of women at risk of familial breast cancer in primary, secondary and tertiary care:

- Women at or near population risk of developing breast cancer (that is, a 10-year risk of less than 3% for women aged 40–49 years and a lifetime risk of less than 17%) are cared for in primary care.
- Women at raised risk of developing breast cancer (that is, a 10-year risk of 3–8% for women aged 40–49 years or a lifetime risk of 17% or greater but less than 30%) are generally cared for in secondary care.
- Women at high risk of developing breast cancer (that is, a 10-year risk of greater than 8% for women aged 40–49 years or a lifetime risk of 30% or greater) are cared for in tertiary care. High risk also includes a 20% or greater chance of a faulty *BRCA1*, *BRCA2* or *TP53* gene in the family.

For the purpose of these calculations, a woman's age should be assumed to be 40 years for a woman in her 40s. A 10-year risk should then be calculated for the age range 40–49 years.

Women who meet the criteria in Box 7 should be offered referral to secondary or tertiary care, as appropriate. NICE has also produced guidelines for mammographic and MRI surveillance (Table 9).

BOX 7. CRITERIA FOR REFERRAL TO SECONDARY AND TERTIARY CARE

Refer to secondary care if:

- one first-degree female relative diagnosed with breast cancer at younger than age 40 years, or
- one first-degree male relative diagnosed with breast cancer at any age, or
- one first-degree relative with bilateral breast cancer where the first primary was diagnosed at younger than age 50 years

or

- two first-degree relatives, or one first-degree and one second-degree relative, diagnosed with breast cancer at any age, or
- one first-degree or second-degree relative diagnosed with breast cancer at any age and one first-degree or second-degree relative diagnosed with ovarian cancer at any age (one of these should be a first-degree relative)

or *(continued on next page)*

- three first-degree or second-degree relatives diagnosed with breast cancer at any age.

Advice should be sought from the designated secondary care contact if any of the following are present in the family history, in addition to breast cancers in relatives not fulfilling the above criteria:

➤ bilateral breast cancer

➤ male breast cancer

➤ ovarian cancer

➤ Jewish ancestry

➤ sarcoma in a relative younger than age 45 years

➤ glioma or childhood adrenal cortical carcinoma

➤ complicated patterns of multiple cancers at a young age

➤ paternal history of breast cancer (two or more relatives on the father's side of the family)

Refer to tertiary care if:

- At least the following female breast cancers only in the family:
  - ◦ two first- or second-degree relatives diagnosed with breast cancer at younger than an average age of 50 years (at least one must be a first-degree relative), or
  - ◦ three first-degree or second-degree relatives diagnosed with breast cancer at younger than an average age of 60 years (at least one must be a first-degree relative), or
  - ◦ four relatives diagnosed with breast cancer at any age (at least one must be a first-degree relative)

or

- Families containing one relative with ovarian cancer at any age and, on the same side of the family:
  - ◦ one first-degree relative (including the relative with ovarian cancer) or second-degree relative diagnosed with breast cancer at younger than age 50 years, or
  - ◦ two first-degree or second-degree relatives diagnosed with breast cancer at younger than an average age of 60 years, or
  - ◦ another ovarian cancer at any age

or

- Families containing bilateral cancer (each breast cancer has the same count value as one relative):
  - ◦ one first-degree relative with cancer diagnosed in both breasts at younger than an average age of 50 years, or *(continued on next page)*

    ○ one first-degree or second-degree relative diagnosed with bilateral breast cancer and one first-degree or second-degree relative diagnosed with breast cancer at younger than an average age of 60 years

or

- Families containing male breast cancer at any age and on the same side of the family, at least:
  - ○ one first-degree or second-degree relative diagnosed with breast cancer at younger than age 50 years, or
  - ○ two first-degree or second-degree relatives diagnosed with breast cancer at younger than an average age of 60 years

or

- A formal risk assessment has given risk estimates of:
  - ○ a 20% or greater chance of a *BRCA1*, *BRCA2* or *TP53* mutation being harboured in the family, or
  - ○ a greater than 8% chance of developing breast cancer age 40–49 years, or
  - ○ a 30% or greater lifetime risk of developing breast cancer

Clinicians should seek further advice from a specialist genetics service for families containing any of the following, in addition to breast cancers:

- ➤ Jewish ancestry
- ➤ sarcoma in a relative younger than age 45 years
- ➤ glioma or childhood adrenal cortical carcinomas
- ➤ complicated patterns of multiple cancers at a young age
- ➤ very strong paternal history (four relatives diagnosed at younger than 60 years of age on the father's side of the family)

All affected relatives must be on the same side of the family and must be blood relatives of the woman and each other.

In cases of bilateral breast cancer, each breast cancer has the same count value as one relative.

Key

First-degree relatives:	Mother, father, daughter, son, sister, brother
Second-degree relatives:	Grandparent, grandchild, aunt, uncle, niece and nephew; half sister and half brother
Third-degree relatives:	Great grandparent, great grandchild, great aunt, great uncle, first cousin, grand nephew and grand niece

Table 9   Guidelines for mammographic and magnetic resonance imaging (MRI) surveillance

Age (years)	Mammography	MRI
20–29	Should not be available for women younger than age 30 years	Should be available only for those at exceptionally high risk (that is, annual risk greater or equal to 1%); for example, *TP53* carriers
30–39	Should be available to women satisfying referral criteria for secondary or specialist care only as part of a research study (ethically approved) or nationally approved and audited service Individualised strategies should be developed for exceptional cases, such as women from families with *BRCA1*, *BRCA1* or *TP53* mutations (or women with equally high risk)	Should be available annually to: • women with a 10-year risk of greater than 8% • *BRCA1*, *BRCA2* or *TP53* mutation carriers • women who have not been tested but have a high chance of carrying a *BRCA1* or *TP53* mutation, specifically: – those at a 50% risk of carrying a *BRCA1* or *TP53* mutation in a tested family – those at 50% risk of carrying a *BRCA1* or *TP53* mutation from untested or inconclusively tested families with at least a 60% risk of a *BRCA1* or *TP53* mutation (that is, a 30% chance of carrying a mutation themselves)
40–49	Should be available annually to women at raised and high risk satisfying referral criteria for secondary or specialist care	Should be available annually to: • women with a 10-year risk of greater than 20% • women with a 10-year risk of greater than 12% whose mammography has shown a dense breast patterna • *TP53*, *BRCA1* and *BRCA21* mutation carriers • Women who have not been tested but have a high chance of carrying a *BRCA1* or *TP53* mutation, specifically: – those at a 50% risk of carrying a *BRCA1* or *TP53* mutation in a tested family – those at 50% risk of carrying a *BRCA1* or *TP53* mutation from untested or inconclusively tested families with at least a 60% risk of a *BRCA1* or *TP53* mutation (that is, a 30% chance of carrying a mutation themselves)

(continued on next page)

Table 9   Guidelines for mammographic and magnetic resonance imaging (MRI) surveillance

Age (years)	Mammography	MRI
50+	Should be available every 3 years as part of the NHS Breast Screening Programme More frequent mammographic surveillance should take place only as part of a research study (ethically approved) or nationally approved and audited service Individualised strategies should be developed for exceptional cases, such as women from families with *BRCA1*, *BRCA2* or *TP53* mutations (or women with equally high risk)	Should not be available for women older than 50 years

[a] As defined by the three-point mammographic classification used by UK breast radiologists (Breast Group of the Royal College of Radiologists 1989)
Supporting information:
An 8% risk aged 30–39 years and a 12% risk aged 40–49 years would be fulfilled by women with the following family histories:
2 close relatives diagnosed with average age < 30 years [b]
3 close relatives diagnosed with average age < 40 years [b]
4 close relatives diagnosed with average age < 50 years [b]
[b] All relatives must be on the same side of the family and one must be a mother or sister of the consultee.
A genetic test would usually be required to determine a 10-year risk of 20% or greater in women aged 40–40 years.
For the purposes of these calculations, a woman's age should be assumed to be 30 years of age for a woman in her 30s and 40 years of age for a woman in her 40s. A 10-year risk should then be calculated for the period 30–39 years and 40–49 years, respectively.

Benign breast disease

Benign breast disease is a generic term describing all non-malignant breast conditions. As such, it encompasses diseases associated with an increased risk of breast cancer and others that do not have a raised risk. Women who have had biopsies that showed proliferative breast disease without atypia have a two-fold increased risk, while women with atypical hyperplasia have a two- to five-fold increased risk.

Although HRT may be associated with mastalgia and promotion of breast cysts, no convincing evidence shows that the risk of breast cancer is increased in women with benign disease. Failure to accurately categorise benign disease, however, prevents determination of whether women involved in these studies were at a significantly increased risk of breast cancer.

Further reading

American Cancer Society. Breast Cancer Facts and Figures 2005–2006 [www.cancer.org/downloads/STT/CAFF2005BrFacspdf2005.pdf].

Anderson GL, Chlebowski RT, Rossouw JE, Rodabough RJ, McTiernan A, Margolis KL, *et al.* Prior hormone therapy and breast cancer risk in the Women's Health Initiative randomized trial of estrogen plus progestin. *Maturitas* 2006;55:103–15.

Banks E, Reeves G, Beral V, Bull D, Crossley B, Simmonds M, *et al.* Impact of use of hormone replacement therapy on false positive recall in the NHS breast screening programme: results from the Million Women Study. *BMJ* 2004;328:1291–2.

Bradbury AR, Olopade OI. Genetic susceptibility to breast cancer. *Rev Endocr Metab Disord* 2007;8(3):255–67.

Cancer research UK [http://info.cancerresearchuk.org/cancerstats/types/breast].

Chlebowski RT, Hendrix SL, Langer RD, Stefanick ML, Gass M, Lane D, *et al.* Influence of estrogen plus progestin on breast cancer and mammography in healthy postmenopausal women. The Women's Health Initiative randomized trial. *JAMA* 2003;289:3243–53.

Collaborative Group on Hormonal Factors in Breast Cancer. Breast Cancer and HRT: collaborative reanalysis of data from 51 epidemiological studies of 52,705 women with breast cancer and 108,411 women without breast cancer. *Lancet* 1997;350:1047–59.

Dimitrakakis C, Jones RA, Liu A, Bondy CA. Breast cancer incidence in postmenopausal women using testosterone in addition to usual hormone therapy. *Menopause* 2004;11(5):531–5.

Dupont WD, Page DL, Parl FF, Plummer WD Jr, Schuyler PA, Kasami M, *et al.* Estrogen replacement therapy in women with a history of proliferative breast disease. *Cancer* 1999;85:1277–83.

Ferlay J, Bray F, Pisani P, Parkin DM. *Globocan 2002: Cancer Incidence, Mortality and Prevalence Worldwide.* Version 2.0. IARC CancerBase no.5. Lyon: IARCPress; 2004.

Greendale GA, Reboussin BA, Slone S, Wasilauskas C, Pike MC, Ursin G. Postmenopausal hormone therapy and change in mammographic density. *J Natl Cancer Inst* 2003;95:30–7.

Holmberg L, Anderson G. HABITS (hormonal replacement therapy after breast cancer: is it safe?), a randomized comparison stopped. *Lancet* 2004;363:453–5.

Kroiss R, Fentiman IS, Helmond FA, Rymer J, Foidart JM, Bundred N, *et al.* The effect of tibolone in postmenopausal women receiving tamoxifen after surgery for breast cancer: a randomised, double-blind, placebo-controlled trial. *BJOG* 2005;112:228–33.

Kwan K, Ward C, Marsden J. Is there a role for hormone replacement therapy after breast cancer? *J Br Menopause Soc* 2005;11:140–4.

McTiernan A, Martin CF, Peck JD, Aragaki AK, Chlebowski RT, Pisano ED, *et al;* Women's Health Initiative Mammogram Density Study Investigators. Estrogen-plus-progestin use and mammographic density in postmenopausal women: women's health initiative randomized trial. *J Natl Cancer Inst* 2005;97:1366–76.

Million Women Study Collaborators. Breast cancer and hormone-replacement therapy in the Million Women Study. *Lancet* 2003;362:419–27.

National Institute for Clinical Excellence. *Familial Breast Cancer.* Clinical Guideline 41. October 2006 [www.nice.org.uk/guidance/cg41].

Office for National Statistics. *Mortality Statistics: Cause. England and Wales 2005.* London TSO; 2006.

Rebbeck TR, Friebel T, Wagner T, Lynch HT, Garber JE, Daly MB, *et al.* Effect of short-term hormone replacement therapy on breast cancer risk reduction after bilateral prophylactic oophorectomy in BRCA1 and BRCA2 mutation carriers: the PROSE Study Group. *J Clin Oncol* 2005;23:7804–10.

Rozenberg S, Antoine C, Carly B, Pastijn A, Liebens F. Improving quality of life after Breast Cancer: prevention of other diseases. *Menopause Int* 2007;13:71–4.

Santen RJ, Mansel R. Benign breast disorders. *N Engl J Med* 2005;353:275–85.

The Women's Health Initiative Steering Committee. Effects of conjugated equine estrogen in postmenopausal women with hysterectomy: the Women's Health Initiative randomized controlled trial. *JAMA* 2004;291:1701–12.

Tamimi RM, Hankinson SE, Chen WY, Rosner B, Colditz GA. Combined estrogen and testosterone use and risk of breast cancer in postmenopausal women. *Arch Intern Med* 2006;166:1483–9.

Von Schoultz E, Rutqvist LE. Menopausal hormone therapy after breast cancer: the Stockholm Randomized Trial. *J Natl Cancer Inst* 2005;97:533–5.

Xydakis AM, Sakkas EG, Mastorakos G. Hormone replacement therapy in breast cancer survivors. *Ann N Y Acad Sci* 2006;1092:349–60.

10 Benign and malignant gynaecological disease

The major concern is the estrogen dependence of these conditions and whether estrogen-based therapy will stimulate growth. Also many treatments for gynaecological cancer may induce a premature menopause resulting in concerns about osteoporosis and cardiovascular disease.

Benign disease

FIBROIDS

Uterine leiomyomas are benign smooth muscle tumours and are the most common gynaecological tumours in women of reproductive age. Uterine leiomyomas clinically affect 25–30% of American women; however, an incidence of 77% has been reported. They are more common in African American women, with some studies indicating they are diagnosed three times more frequently than in white women. They are often associated with reproductive and gynaecological disorders ranging from infertility and pregnancy loss to pelvic pain and excessive uterine bleeding. They are steroid-dependent tumours that rarely progress to malignancy and regress at the menopause.

There is a concern that they may become enlarged with estrogen treatment and cause heavy or painful withdrawal bleeds, so the woman should be advised of this. The evidence of the effect of different types of HRT, including tibolone, on fibroid growth is poor. Ultrasound examinations may be helpful in documenting the fibroids and, if clinically indicated, regular pelvic examinations are recommended. Limited data suggest that raloxifene shrinks fibroids.

ENDOMETRIOSIS

Endometriosis is defined as endometrium in sites other than the uterine cavity; this ectopic endometrium undergoes a similar morphological pattern to the eutopic (normally placed) endometrium during the menstrual cycle. This is another steroid-dependent condition. It is found in around 10% of women of reproductive age and in up to 25% of women undergoing hysterectomy. It is a difficult management problem, as estrogen can theoretically reactivate the disease, even when the woman has had apparent surgical removal of all the endometriotic tissue. Concerns are disease recurrence and malignant changes arising from the presence of residual endometriosis. The risks are small and the evidence base of various strategies is poor.

Women with a history of endometriosis may be at particular risk of the long-term consequences of estrogen deficiency as a consequence of repeated courses of gonadotrophin hormone-releasing analogues or premature surgical menopause. Some gynaecologists avoid starting estrogen-based HRT for the first 6 months after oophorectomy, preferring to give a progestogen alone, continuous combined therapy or tibolone to control hot flushes when the woman has extensive disease. No good evidence base is available on whether to recommend an unopposed regimen, an opposed continuous combined regimen or tibolone. Management of potential recurrence is best monitored by responding to the recurrence of symptoms. Limited data suggest that raloxifene is not helpful in the treatment of endometriosis and there is no information regarding its use in menopausal women with a history of endometriosis. The effects of phytoestrogens or herbal preparations on ectopic endometrium are uncertain.

Gynaecological cancer

In the USA, there were 71 090 new cases of gynaecological cancer in 2006. Ovarian, cervical, vaginal and vulval cancer are not estrogen-dependent conditions and estrogen replacement is not contraindicated. However, there is some doubt with regard to endometrioid ovarian cancer and endometrial carcinoma is often listed in data sheets as an absolute contraindication to HRT. There is a paucity of information about the use of tibolone or raloxifene after gynaecological cancer. The safety of alternative and complementary therapies is unknown.

OVARIAN CANCER

HRT and ovarian cancer risk

This is an area where there is considerable uncertainty. Meta-analyses have produced conflicting results with one showing a summary relative risk of 1.15 (95% CI 1.05–1.27) and another concluding that there was no statistically significant association between ever and never use (odds ratio 1.1; 95% CI 0.9–1.3) nor any evident dose–response relationship. However, prospective studies have suggested a modest effect after long-term use such as 10 or more years. The randomised WHI found no significant increase with combined estrogen–progestogen HRT. The observational MWS also found a small increase, namely that HRT taken over 5 years resulted in one extra ovarian cancer in roughly 2500 HRT users and one extra ovarian cancer death in roughly 3300 users. HRT use does not appear to adversely influence the risk of ovarian cancer in *BRCA1* and *BRCA2* mutation carriers.

HRT after ovarian cancer
Studies of estrogen replacement do not show a detrimental effect on survival. They are mainly observational. There is a paucity of data regarding endometrioid ovarian cancer. Its potential estrogen dependence intuitively leads to the use of combined estrogen–progestogen HRT rather than estrogen alone. The rationale of progestogen addition is to suppress any estrogen-stimulated growth.

Prophylactic oophorectomy
Bilateral prophylactic oophorectomy is increasingly being performed in women at high risk of ovarian cancer such as *BRCA1* and *BRCA2* mutation carriers. The average cumulative risk by age 70 years has been estimated to be 39% (18–54%) in *BRCA1* mutation carriers and 11% (2.4–19%) for *BRCA2*. Data regarding HRT use after prophylactic oophorectomy are limited and show no adverse effect.

ENDOMETRIAL CANCER

HRT and endometrial cancer risk
Unopposed estrogen replacement therapy increases endometrial cancer risk. Most studies have shown that this excess risk is not completely eliminated with monthly sequential progestogen addition, especially when continued for more than 5 years. This has also been found with long-cycle HRT. No increased risk of endometrial cancer has been found with continuous combined regimens. Raloxifene does not stimulate the endometrium and there is no increased of endometrial cancer. While observational studies have suggested that tibolone increases the risk of endometrial cancer this has not been confirmed in RCTs.

HRT after endometrial cancer
Previous endometrial carcinoma often is listed in datasheets as an absolute contraindication to estrogen replacement therapy; however, no data show an increased risk of recurrence or mortality. On the contrary, a reduction in frequency of relapses is shown together with longer disease-free intervals and also longer survival times. A systematic review concluded that there seems to be no indication for adjuvant progestogens after early stage endometrial cancer. Progestogens, however, do play a role in women with advanced or recurrent disease. Thus, use of HRT in endometrial cancer survivors especially in stage I or II disease is not contraindicated.

CERVICAL CANCER

Cervical cancer is not an estrogen-dependent disease and so HRT is not contraindicated. In women who have had a hysterectomy, estrogen only can be used. However, in those treated by radiotherapy and in whom the uterus is retained it cannot be assumed that all the endometrium has been destroyed. Indeed, there are reports of endometrial cancers developing after definitive radiation treatment for invasive cervical cancer. In women who retain their uterus a progestogen must be added to the estrogen.

Further reading

BENIGN DISEASE

Bain C. Managing women with a previous diagnosis of endometriosis. *J Br Menopause Soc* 2006;12:28–33.

Dixon D, Parrott EC, Segars JH, Olden K, Pinn VW. The second National Institutes of Health International Congress on advances in uterine leiomyoma research: conference summary and future recommendations. *Fertil Steril* 2006;86:800–6.

Fedele L, Bianchi S, Raffaelli R, Zanconato G. A randomized study of the effects of tibolone and transdermal estrogen replacement therapy in postmenopausal women with uterine myomas. *Eur J Obstet Gynecol Reprod Biol* 2000;88:91–4.

Guo SW, Olive DL. Two Unsuccessful Clinical Trials on Endometriosis and a Few Lessons Learned. *Gynecol Obstet Invest* 2007;64:24–35.

Lingxia X, Taixiang W, Xiaoyan C. Selective estrogen receptor modulators (SERMs) for uterine leiomyomas. *Cochrane Database Syst Rev* 2007;(2):CD005287.

Matorras R, Elorriaga MA, Pijoan JI, Ramón O, Rodríguez-Escudero FJ. Recurrence of endometriosis in women with bilateral adnexectomy (with or without total hysterectomy) who received hormone replacement therapy. *Fertil Steril* 2002;77:303–8.

Morrison J, MacKenzie IZ. Uterine fibroids. In: *The Abnormal Menstrual Cycle.* Rees M, Hope S, Ravnikar V, editors. Abingdon: Taylor and Francis; 2005. p.79–93.

Palomba S, Orio F Jr, Russo T, Falbo A, Tolino A, Lombardi G, *et al.* Antiproliferative and proapoptotic effects of raloxifene on uterine leiomyomas in postmenopausal women. *Fertil Steril* 2005;84:154–61.

GYNAECOLOGICAL CANCER

Anderson GL, Judd HL, Kaunitz AM, Barad DH, Beresford SA, Pettinger M, *et al;* Women's Health Initiative Investigators. Effects of estrogen plus progestin on gynecologic cancers and associated diagnostic procedures: the Women's Health Initiative randomized trial. *JAMA* 2003;290:1739–48.

American Cancer Society. Cancer Facts and Figures 2006. [www.cancer.org/downloads/STT/CAFF2006PWSecured.pdf].

Rees M. Gynaecological oncology perspective on management of the menopause. *Eur J Surg Oncol* 2006;32:892–7.

OVARIAN CANCER

Antoniou A, Pharoah PD, Narod S, Risch HA, Eyfjord JE, Hopper JL, *et al.* Average risks of breast and ovarian cancer associated with *BRCA1* or *BRCA2* mutations detected in case series unselected for family history: a combined analysis of 22 studies. *Am J Hum Genet* 2003;72:1117–30.

Beral V; Million Women Study Collaborators, Bull D, Green J, Reeves G. Ovarian cancer and hormone replacement therapy in the Mmillion Women Study. *Lancet* 2007;369:1703–10.

Coughlin SS, Giustozzi A, Smith SJ, Lee NC. A meta-analysis of estrogen replacement therapy and risk of epithelial ovarian cancer. *J Clin Epidemiol* 2000;53:367–75.

Garg PP, Kerlikowske K, Subak L, Grady D. Hormone replacement therapy and the risk of epithelial ovarian carcinoma: a meta-analysis. *Obstet Gynecol* 1998;92:472–9.

Kotsopoulos J, Lubinski J, Neuhausen SL, Lynch HT, Rosen B, Ainsworth P, *et al.* Hormone replacement therapy and the risk of ovarian cancer in *BRCA1* and *BRCA2* mutation carriers. *Gynecol Oncol* 2006;100:83–8.

Lacey JV Jr, Brinton LA, Leitzmann MF, Mouw T, Hollenbeck A, Schatzkin A, *et al.* Menopausal hormone therapy and ovarian cancer risk in the National Institutes of Health-AARP Diet and Health Study Cohort. *J Natl Cancer Inst* 2006;98:1397–405.

Mascarenhas C, Lambe M, Bellocco R, Bergfeldt K, Riman T, Persson I, *et al.* Use of hormone replacement therapy before and after ovarian cancer diagnosis and ovarian cancer survival. *Int J Cancer* 2006;119:2907–15.

Riman T. Hormone replacement therapy and epithelial ovarian cancer: is there an association? *J Br Menopause Soc* 2003;9:61–8.

Rodriguez C, Patel AV, Calle EE, Jacob EJ, Thun MJ. Estrogen replacement therapy and ovarian cancer mortality in a large prospective study of US women. *JAMA* 2001;285:1460–5.

Ursic-Vrscaj M, Bebar S, Zakelj MP. Hormone replacement therapy after invasive ovarian serous cystadenocarcinoma treatment: the effect on survival. *Menopause* 2001;8:70–5.

ENDOMETRIAL CANCER

Archer DF, Hendrix S, Gallagher JC, Rymer J, Skouby S, Ferenczy A, *et al.* Endometrial effects of tibolone. *J Clin Endocrinol Metab* 2007;92:911–18.

Beral V, Bull D, Reeves G; Million Women Study Collaborators. Endometrial cancer and hormone-replacement therapy in the Million Women Study. *Lancet* 2005;365:1543–51.

Grady D, Ettinger B, Moscarelli E, Plouffe L Jr, Sarkar S, Ciaccia A, *et al;* Multiple Outcomes of Raloxifene Evaluation Investigators. Safety and adverse effects associated with raloxifene: multiple outcomes of raloxifene evaluation. *Obstet Gynecol* 2004;104:837–44.

Martin-Hirsch PL, Jarvis G, Kitchener H, Lilford R. Progestogens for endometrial cancer. *Cochrane Database Syst Rev* 2000:(2)CD001040.

Suriano KA, McHale M, McLaren CE, Li KT, Re A, DiSaia PJ. Estrogen replacement therapy in endometrial cancer patients: a matched control study. *Obstet Gynecol* 2001;97:955–60.

Weiderpass E, Adami HO, Baron JA, Magnusson C, Bergström R, Lindgren A, *et al.* Risk of endometrial cancer following estrogen replacement with and without progestins. *J Natl Cancer Inst* 1999;91:1131–7.

CERVICAL CANCER

Pothuri B, Ramondetta L, Martino M, Alektiar K, Eifel PJ, Deavers MT, *et al.* Development of endometrial cancer after radiation treatment for cervical carcinoma. *Obstet Gynecol* 2003;101:941–5.

11 Premature menopause

The terms 'premature menopause' or 'premature ovarian failure' describe a stop in the normal functioning of the ovaries in a woman younger than age 40 years. The condition is common. Overall, premature ovarian failure is responsible for 4–18% of cases of secondary amenorrhoea and 10–28% of primary amenorrhoea. It is estimated to affect 1% of women younger than 40 years and 0.1% of those under 30 years. It is important to note that, unless the woman has undergone bilateral oophorectomy, menstruation can recommence and spontaneous pregnancy may still occur.

Symptoms and health consequences of premature ovarian failure

The most common first symptom of premature ovarian failure is irregular periods. Others may present through infertility services. Some women with premature ovarian failure also have other symptoms, similar to those of women with ovarian failure in their 50s. These may include:

- hot flushes and night sweats
- irritability, poor concentration
- decreased libido and dyspareunia
- vaginal dryness.

Mean life expectancy in women with menopause before the age of 40 years is 2.0 years shorter than that in women with menopause after the age of 55 years. Women with untreated premature menopause are at increased risk of developing osteoporosis, cardiovascular disease, dementia, cognitive decline and parkinsonism but at lower risk of breast malignancy. Premature menopause can lead to reduced peak bone mass (if the woman is younger than 25 years) or early bone loss thereafter. The increased risk of coronary heart disease has been noted especially in smokers.

Premature ovarian failure frequently is associated with autoimmune disorders, particularly hypothyroidism (25%), Addison's disease (3%) and diabetes mellitus (2.5%). It is important that these diseases should be screened for in women with primary premature ovarian failure.

Aetiology

PRIMARY PREMATURE OVARIAN FAILURE

Primary premature ovarian failure can occur at any age, even in teenagers. It can present as primary or secondary amenorrhoea. Traditional texts have distinguished between follicular depletion and dysfunction. In the absence of noninvasive tests to differentiate between the two, the only alternative is laparoscopic ovarian biopsy. However, validity of single biopsies has been questioned, with pregnancies occurring despite lack of follicles in the biopsy material. About 10–20% of women with premature ovarian failure have a family history of the condition. This finding suggests that some cases of premature ovarian failure can be genetic. However, genetics is not the only cause of premature ovarian failure. In the great majority of cases, no cause can be found.

Chromosome abnormalities

A critical region on the X-chromosome (POF1), which ranges from Xq13 to Xq26, which relates to normal ovarian function has been identified, as has a second gene of paternal origin (POF2), which is located at Xq13.3–q21.1. Idiopathic premature ovarian failure can be familial or sporadic and the familial pattern of inheritance is compatible with X-linked with incomplete penetrance or an autosomal dominant mode of inheritance. In Turner syndrome, complete absence of one X chromosome (45XO) results in ovarian dysgenesis and primary ovarian failure. Familial premature ovarian failure has been linked with fragile X permutations. Fragile X mutations occur at least ten times more often in women with premature ovarian failure than the general population. Women with Down syndrome (trisomy 21) also have an early menopause. The BEPS (benign edematous polysynovitis syndrome) is a rare autosomal dominant condition that leads to congenital abnormalities of the eye, including blepharophimosis, ptosis and epicanthus inversis. In BEPS I, eyelid malformation cosegregates with premature ovarian failure and has been mapped to chromosome 3q.17.

Follicle-stimulating hormone receptor gene polymorphism and inhibin B mutation

Resistance to the action of gonadotrophins can lead to the clinical features of premature ovarian failure and this has been shown in a cohort of Finnish families. This is a very rare cause. In addition, a mutation in the inhibin gene that has a frequency ten-fold higher than in control women (7.0% versus 0.7%) has been identified.

Enzyme deficiencies

A number of enzyme deficiencies have been found to be associated with an increased risk of premature ovarian failure. The most common of these is the autosomal recessive condition of galactosaemia, in which there is a deficiency in the enzyme galactose-1-phosphate uridyltransferase. Other enzyme abnormalities associated with premature ovarian failure include deficiencies of 17_-hydroxylase, 17-20 desmolase and cholesterol desmolase. Deficiency of 17_-hydroxylase can prevent estradiol synthesis, which leads to primary amenorrhoea and elevated levels of gonadotrophins, even though developing follicles are present.

Women with a deficiency of cholesterol desmolase are not able to produce biologically active steroids and rarely survive to adulthood.

Autoimmune disease
Premature ovarian failure frequently is associated with autoimmune disorders such as:

- hypothyroidism
- Addison's disease
- diabetes mellitus
- Crohn's disease
- vitiligo
- pernicious anaemia
- systemic lupus erythematosus
- rheumatoid arthritis.

Addison's disease may be present as part of a polyglandular failure syndrome. The type I syndrome is associated with premature ovarian failure. It comprises adrenal failure, hypoparathyroidism and chronic mucocutaneous candidiasis and mainly occurs in children. The type II syndrome may present much later with hypothyroidism and is less consistently associated with premature ovarian failure.

Circulating antiovarian antibodies have been found in 10–69% of women with premature ovarian failure but also in a significant number of controls. Anti-gonadotrophin receptor antibodies have been isolated but their significance remains unclear. Antibodies directed against steroid-producing cells have proved most promising in terms of predicting which women may develop ovarian failure as part of the polyglandular syndrome but these are found in a minority of those with premature ovarian failure.

SECONDARY PREMATURE OVARIAN FAILURE

Secondary premature ovarian failure is becoming more important, as survival after the treatment of malignancy continues to improve. The development of techniques to conserve ovarian tissue or oocytes before therapy is instigated should help with maintenance of fertility. The causes of secondary premature ovarian failure are detailed below.

Chemotherapy and radiotherapy

The likelihood of ovarian failure after chemotherapy or radiotherapy depends on the agent used, dosage levels, interval between treatments and, particularly, the age of the woman, which probably reflects the age-related progressive natural decline in the oocyte pool. The prepubertal ovary is relatively resistant to the effects of chemotherapeutic alkylating agents. Attempts to suppress the ovarian activity of women of reproductive age with oral contraceptives or gonadotrophin hormone-releasing analogues in order to mimic this protection have produced conflicting results.

Radiation-induced ovarian failure usually results in sterility when the total dose exceeds 6 Gy. As with chemotherapy, however, prepubertal girls are more resistant to irradiation. Normal menstruation after treatment does not necessarily mean that the ovaries are unaffected and premature menopause can occur, resulting in a shorter reproductive span. Surgical transposition of the ovaries outside of the direct field of treatment has been described. High-dose pelvic radiotherapy will have long-term effects on the uterine vasculature and development. Adverse pregnancy outcomes include an increased risk of early pregnancy loss, preterm birth and delivery of infants with low or very low birth weights.

Bilateral oophorectomy

This results in an immediate menopause. The implications of this procedure require detailed preoperative discussion.

Hysterectomy without oophorectomy

This can induce ovarian failure in the immediate postoperative period, where in some cases it may be temporary, or at a later stage, where it may occur sooner than the time of natural menopause. This is an area of controversy and may depend on ovarian function preceding hysterectomy. It is essential to counsel women about this preoperatively. The diagnosis may be difficult, as not all women have hot flushes and, in the absence of a uterus, the pointer of amenorrhoea is absent. A case could be made for annual estimates of levels of FSH in women who have had a hysterectomy before the age of 40 years.

Infection

Tuberculosis and mumps are infections that have been implicated most commonly. In most cases, normal ovarian function returns after infection with mumps. Malaria, varicella and shigella infections have also been implicated in premature ovarian failure.

Investigations

Investigation of premature menopause are:

- estimates of levels of FSH in serum (x 2)
- thyroid function tests
- autoimmune screen for polyendocrinopathy
- chromosome analysis, especially in women younger than 30 years
- estimates of bone mineral density through DXA (optional)
- adrenocorticotrophic hormone stimulation test if Addison's disease is suspected (optional).

The diagnostic usefulness of ovarian biopsy outside the context of a research setting has yet to be proved. Assessment of ovarian reserve is a controversial area. Parameters of ovarian reserve that have been studied include FSH, luteinising hormone (LH), estradiol, inhibin B, anti-müllerian hormone, total antral follicle count and ovarian volume. As yet, no single clinically useful test is available to predict ovarian reserve accurately and a combination of markers ultimately may be more helpful.

Premature ovarian failure, fertility and contraception

Women with premature ovarian failure are unlikely to become spontaneously pregnant. There is no proven treatment to improve a woman's ability to have a baby naturally. However, the lifetime chance of spontaneous conception in women with karyotypically normal premature ovarian failure has been estimated at 5–15%, with the age of the woman at the time of diagnosis being an important determinant. Donor oocyte *in vitro* fertilisation (IVF) is the treatment of choice. Women with spontaneous, karyotypically normal premature ovarian failure have similar success rates to women who undergo conventional IVF. The age of the oocyte rather than the age of the recipient determines the chance of success. Oocyte donation also is an option for women with Turner syndrome and pregnancy rates in observational studies are similar to those with oocyte donation for other indications. The risk of miscarriage, however, is greater. Cardiovascular and other complications, such as hypertension and pre-eclampsia, occur more frequently in women with Turner syndrome.

Very few options are available for preventative therapy before radiotherapy and chemotherapy. Mature oocytes and ovarian tissue cannot be cryopreserved easily; however, successful pregnancies have been achieved. The collection of mature oocytes requires ovarian stimulation, which may not be advisable in women with estrogen-dependent malignancies. In addition, these techniques are not suitable for prepubertal women. Cryopreservation of embryos may be possible before treatment – if time allows and fertility drugs are not contraindicated.

If the woman does not want to have further children she would need to consider continuing an effective form of contraception. The levonorgestrel-releasing intrauterine contraceptive device would also provide the progestogen component of a HRT regimen (see Chapter 3). Elevated FSH levels do not mean that a woman is infertile. The next decision will be duration of contraception. Traditionally, women have been advised that contraception can be stopped if they have been amenorrhoeic for 2 years before the age of 50 years and 1 year above that. However, the menstrual pattern will be difficult to establish if she is using HRT or the levonorgestrel-releasing intrauterine contraceptive device and she could be advised to continue with contraception until the age of 55 years.

Hormone replacement therapy

Estrogen replacement therapy is the mainstay of treatment for women with premature ovarian failure and is recommended until the average age of natural menopause. This view is endorsed by national and international regulatory bodies. There is no evidence that estrogen replacement increases the risk of breast cancer to a level greater than that found in normally menstruating women and women with premature ovarian failure do not need to start mammographic screening early. HRT or the combined estrogen and progestogen contraceptive pill may be used. The latter has the psychological benefit of being a treatment used by many of the woman's peer group and this is important when dealing with young women or teenagers. Women with premature ovarian failure who take HRT may need a higher dose of estrogen to control vasomotor symptoms than women in their 50s.

No clinical trial evidence attests the efficacy or safety of the use of non-estrogen-based treatments, such as bisphosphonates, strontium ranelate or raloxifene, in these women. Their effects on the developing fetal skeleton are unknown.

Some women complain of reduced libido or sexual function despite apparently adequate doses of estrogen replacement. Testosterone should be considered and a testosterone patch for female use is now available.

Counselling

Women who suffer from premature ovarian failure must be provided with adequate information. They may find it a difficult diagnosis to accept, especially if they wish to have children. National self-support groups for premature ovarian failure exist and these provide helpful psychological support for many women.

Further reading

Beerendonk CC, Braat DD. Present and future options for the preservation of fertility in female adolescents with cancer. *Endocr Dev* 2005;8:166–75.

Donnez J, Dolmans MM, Demylle D, Jadoul P, Pirard C, Squifflet J, *et al.* Livebirth after orthotopic transplantation of cryopreserved ovarian tissue. *Lancet* 2004;364:1405–10.

Ewertz M, Mellemkjaer L, Poulsen AH, Friis S, Sørensen HT, Pedersen L, *et al.* Hormone use for menopausal symptoms and risk of breast cancer. A Danish cohort study. *Br J Cancer* 2005;92:1293–7.

Faculty of Family Planning and Reproductive Health Care. Clinical Effectiveness Unit. Contraception for women aged over 40 years. *J Fam Plann Reprod Health Care* 2005;31:51–64.

Farquhar CM, Sadler L, Harvey SA, Stewart AW. The association of hysterectomy and menopause: a prospective cohort study. *BJOG* 2005;112:956–62.

Groff AA, Covington SN, Halverson LR, Fitzgerald OR, Vanderhoof V, Calis K, *et al.* Assessing the emotional needs of women with spontaneous premature ovarian failure. *Fertil Steril* 2005;83:1734–41.

Jacobsen BK, Knutsen SF, Fraser GE. Age at natural menopause and total mortality and mortality from ischemic heart disease: the Adventist Health Study. *J Clin Epidemiol* 1999;52:303–7.

Lutchman Singh K, Davies M, Chatterjee R. Fertility in female cancer survivors: pathophysiology, preservation and the role of ovarian reserve testing. *Hum Reprod Update* 2005;11:69–89.

National Collaborating Centre for Women's and Children's Health. *Fertility: Assessment and Treatment for People with Fertility Problems.* London: RCOG Press; 2004. p. 126–7.

Nelson LM, Covington SN, Rebar RW. An update: spontaneous premature ovarian failure is not an early menopause. *Fertil Steril* 2005;83:1327–32.

Ossewaarde ME, Bots ML, Verbeek AL, Peeters PH, van der Graaf Y, Grobbee DE, *et al.* Age at menopause, cause-specific mortality and total life expectancy. *Epidemiology* 2005;16:556–62.

Pitkin J, Rees MCP, Gray S, Lumsden MA, Marsden J, Stevenson JC, *et al.* British Menopause Society Council Consensus Statement. Management of premature menopause. *Menopause Int* 2007;13:44–45.

Rocca WA, Grossardt BR, de Andrade M, Malkasian GD, Melton LJ 3rd. Survival patterns after oophorectomy in premenopausal women: a population-based cohort study. *Lancet Oncol* 2006;7:821–8.

Rocca WA, Bower JH, Maraganore DM, Ahlskog JE, Grossardt BR, de Andrade M, *et al.* Increased risk of cognitive impairment or dementia in women who underwent oophorectomy before menopause. *Neurology* 2007;691074–83.

Rocca WA, Bower JH, Maraganore DM, Ahlskog JE, Grossardt BR, de Andrade M, Melton LJ 3rd. Increased risk of parkinsonism in women who underwent oophorectomy before menopause. *Neurology* 2008;70:200–9.

Shifren JL, Davis SR, Moreau M, Waldbaum A, Bouchard C, DeRogatis L, *et al.* Testosterone patch for the treatment of hypoactive sexual desire disorder in naturally menopausal women: results from the INTIMATE NM1 Study. *Menopause* 2006;13:770–9.

Tucker D. Premature ovarian failure. In: Rees M, Hope S, Ravnikar V. *The Abnormal Menstrual Cycle*. Abingdon: Taylor and Francis; 2005. p. 111–22.

Wallace WH, Thomson AB, Saran F, Kelsey TW. Predicting age of ovarian failure after radiation to a field that includes the ovaries. *Int J Radiat Oncol Biol Phys* 2005;62:738–44.

12 Women with concomitant medical problems

Cardiovascular disease

Cardiovascular disease, of which coronary heart disease (CHD) and stroke are the primary clinical endpoints, is the leading cause of death in older women (Table 10). Although cardiovascular disease is rarely the cause of death in women before the sixth decade, it is the most common cause after the age of 60 years. Whereas menopause, of itself, has not been thought of as being the specific cause of cardiovascular disease in women, certain risk factors increase after menopause, which may help explain the exaggerated increase in its incidence after menopause. These include an accelerated rise in cholesterol levels, blood pressure and insulin resistance, primarily with increasing body weight. Mortality rates may be increased in women with early menopause, either spontaneous or surgically induced.

CORONARY HEART DISEASE

CHD by itself is the most common cause of death in the UK. Around one in five men and one in six women die from the disease. CHD causes around 106 000 deaths in the UK each year. Women share the same

Age (years)	Coronary heart disease		Stroke	
	Men	Women	Men	Women
All ages	58,555	47,287	22,970	37,488
< 35	136	36	109	100
35–44	850	196	263	207
45–54	3,041	610	613	530
55–64	7,369	2,006	1,434	1,085
65–74	14,149	6,634	3,955	3,289
≤ 75	33,010	37,805	16,596	32,277

Table 10 Deaths by cause, sex and age, 2004, UK (Sources: Office for National Statistics; General Register Office, Edinburgh; General Register Office, Northern Ireland)

cardiovascular risk factors as men and diabetes confers the maximal additional risk. Women tend to be 8–10 years older than men at presentation – a factor that may influence therapeutic decisions and responses to treatment. Women present with different symptoms from men particularly in terms of acute coronary syndromes such as myocardial infraction and unstable angina leading to delays in diagnosis.

Coronary heart disease and HRT

There is an overwhelming body of evidence from observational studies that women who take HRT have a lower risk of CHD than non-users. This was found for both opposed and unopposed estrogen. However, this has not been borne out in randomised primary and secondary prevention RCTs (Table 11). The role of HRT in primary or secondary prevention thus now is uncertain and it should not be used primarily for this indication at this time.

The timing, dose and possibly type of HRT, however, may be critical in determining cardiovascular effects, as found in the WHI and prospective cohort Nurses' Health Study. Women in the WHI who started combined HRT within 10 years of the menopause had a lower risk of CHD than women who started later (see Chapter 2).

STROKE

The incidence of stroke increases with age, doubling in each decade of life after the sixth decade (Table 10). One in five 50-year-old white women in the Western world will experience a stroke during their lifetime. Many

Table 11. The principle randomised trial results on the end points of stroke or myocardial infarction (source: Lloyd, 2007)

Study acronym	HRT type	Target prevention population	Number	MI (% change in risk)	Stroke (% change in risk)
WHI	CEE/MPA	Primary	16608	29	41
WHI (E)	CEE	Primary	10739	–11	39
HERS	CEE/MPA	Secondary	2763	–1	NS
HERS II	CEE/MPA	Secondary	2763	0	NS
ESPRIT	Estradiol valerate	Secondary	1017	0	36
WEST	17β-estradiol oral	Secondary	664	10	0
PHASE	17β-estradiol patch	Secondary	255	29	NS

NS not studied, CEE = conjugated equine estrogens, MI = myocardial infarction, MPA = medroxyprogesterone acetate survivors are left with significant physical and mental impairment and have serious long-term disability. The most common form of stroke involves brain ischaemia resulting from obstruction of the cerebral arteries. Other forms of stroke involve the rupture of aneurysms leading to primary intracerebral and subarachnoid haemorrhage.

Stroke and HRT

A substantial body of observational data is available on HRT and stroke. Interpretation is complicated, however, by the differences in study design, failure to differentiate between ischaemic and haemorrhagic stroke and the status of HRT use (current users versus ever users). The observational Nurses' Health Study showed no increase in the incidence of stroke except when high-dose estrogen was used. Similarly, the randomised HERS study found no increase in stroke.

Both the estrogen alone and the combined arms of WHI found an increase in ischaemic but not haemorrhagic stroke. The excess absolute risk for the combined HRT arm was four cases of stroke/10 000 women/year at 50–59 years, nine at 60–69 years and 13 at 70–79 years. The excess absolute risk for the estrogen-alone arm was 0 cases of stroke/10 000 women/year at 50–59 years, 19 at 60–69 years and 14 at 70–79 years. When the two arms were combined risk did not vary significantly by age or time since menopause.

In women who have already experienced a previous ischaemic stroke, estrogen replacement does not reduce mortality or recurrence, as evidenced by data from RCTs. Tibolone increases the risk of stroke.

HYPERTENSION

There is no evidence that estradiol-based HRT increases blood pressure or has an adverse effect in women with hypertension. Rarely, conjugated equine estrogens may cause severe hypertension that returns to normal when treatment is stopped. Data from trials of tibolone and raloxifene do not show an adverse effect on blood pressure.

VALVULAR HEART DISEASE

HRT is not contraindicated in women with valvular heart disease. Women who take anticoagulants may have more problems with irregular or heavy bleeding, which requires an adjustment of the dose of progestogen relative to that of the estrogen. Endometrial biopsy, if required, should be performed under antibiotic cover.

HYPERLIPIDAEMIA

Various lipid and lipoprotein profiles increase the risk of cardiovascular disease. The most significant are high-density lipoprotein C (HDL-C), triglyceride and lipoprotein(a). The increased risk associated with increased levels of triglycerides and low-density lipoprotein C (LDL-C) can be offset by increased levels of HDL-C. In terms of lipids, the ideal HRT would increase HDL-C without increasing triglyceride and decrease LDL-C and lipoprotein(a). The effects depend on the type of steroid and the route of administration and HRT can be tailored to the lipid profile.

Oral estrogen reduces lipoprotein(a) and LDL-C and increases HDL-C and triglycerides. Transdermal estrogen does not increase triglycerides or HDL-C but is less effective at reducing lipoprotein(a) and LDL-C. Oral HRT with a non-androgenic progestogen (dydrogesterone) will increase HDL-C and triglycerides and decrease LDL-C and lipoprotein(a). Oral HRT with a 19-nortestosterone (norethisterone) derivative will decrease LDL-C and lipoprotein(a) but will not increase HDL and will be neutral for triglycerides. Thus, in women with hypertriglyceridaemia, the transdermal route is preferred to the oral route. Hormone replacement therapy can be combined with statins.

Raloxifene and tamoxifen reduce levels of total cholesterol and LDL-C while remaining neutral towards triglyceride and HDL-C. However a large randomised trial (RUTH) found that raloxifene did not reduce the risk of CHD.

VENOUS THROMBOEMBOLISM

HRT increases the risk of venous thromboembolism (VTE). The randomised Heart and Estrogen/progestin Replacement Study (HERS) and WHI found that for combined therapy, the odds ratio was 2.7 (1.4–5.0) in HERS and 2.1 (1.6–2.7) in WHI. The highest risk occurs in the first year of use. The absolute risk is small, however, as VTE occurs in 1.7/1000 in women older than 50 years who are not taking HRT and mortality is low (1–2%). Advancing age, obesity and an underlying thrombophilia, such as factor V Leiden, significantly increase risk. For example, in the placebo arm of the WHI, the number of cases of VTE/1000 women/year was 0.8 at 50–59 years, 1.9 at 60–69 years and 2.7 at 70–79 years. While raloxifene and progestogens in non-contraceptive doses increase the risk of VTE, little is known about the effect of tibolone.

HRT after VTE

A history of VTE is the biggest risk factor for future VTE and is a relative contraindication to HRT. In women who have taken estrogen-based HRT after VTE, data from randomised trials show an increased risk of recurrence in the first year of use. It is essential to confirm whether any personal event has been confirmed objectively and what was the severity of the episode. After a single episode of VTE, a constant risk of recurrence of 5% per year exists when anticoagulation is discontinued.

If it is thought that the benefits of HRT outweigh the risks for a particular individual, such as a woman with a premature menopause, a thrombophilia screen then may be justified, as the finding of a severe defect or a combination of defects might alter the perceived risk–benefit assessment. A negative thrombophilia screen must not be used to give false reassurance. The woman may be at high risk, even though no pathological explanation is present. Women older than 50 years with a history of VTE within the previous year, in addition to thrombophilia screening, should be screened for underlying disease, including malignancy and connective tissue disorders.

If HRT is used, the transdermal route might be safer and raloxifene, progestogens and tibolone are best avoided (see above). Norpregnane progestogens may be thrombogenic, whereas micronised progesterone and pregnane derivatives appear safe with respect to thrombotic risk.

In women on long-term warfarin, HRT, raloxifene, progestogens and tibolone can be prescribed, as the risk of recurrence should be very small provided anticoagulation continues. However, anticoagulation to allow HRT use is rarely a good option as about one in 400 patients on warfarin bleed to death each year.

HRT and a family history of thrombosis

Testing for hereditary thrombophilia must be undertaken in conjunction with taking a detailed family history. Again, a negative thrombophilia screen must not be used to give false reassurance if there is a significant family history. With regard to treatment, transdermal estrogen might be safer and raloxifene, progestogens and tibolone are best avoided.

Endocrine disorders

DIABETES MELLITUS

Diabetes mellitus is one of the most common endocrine disorders and it affects almost 6% of the world population. The number of diabetic patients has been estimated to reach 300 million in 2025. More than 97% of these patients will have type 2 diabetes. Obesity is a major risk factor and this is of paramount importance with the obesity epidemic in developed countries. HRT may decrease the incidence of type 2 diabetes mellitus, as well as improving glycaemic control, with results varying according to the type and route of administration. It also improves lipid profiles and transdermal delivery seems to decrease triglyceride levels. Data on the effect of HRT on CHD are conflicting; however, it might be beneficial in younger women with postmenopausal diabetes, whereas it cannot be advised for women older than 60 years with, or at high risk of, cardiovascular disease. Cardioprotective adjunctive treatments (such as statins or low-dose aspirin) can be prescribed concomitantly with HRT. Osteoporosis is reported as a potential complication of type 1 diabetes mellitus but the effects of type 2 diabetes mellitus on bone mass are conflicting. Both type 1 and 2 diabetes increase the risk of endometrial cancer and thus diabetic women must receive a progestogen if the uterus is intact. Little is known about the use of either raloxifene or tibolone in diabetic women.

THYROID DISEASE

Thyroid dysfunction is common in the general population, especially among older women. Estimates of prevalence vary but up to 20% of women may be affected. Postmenopausal women are at increased risk for both osteoporosis and cardiovascular disease. Undiagnosed and untreated thyroid disease may exacerbate these risks. A past history of hyperthyroidism of any aetiology is associated with an increased risk of osteoporosis and hip fracture, particularly in postmenopausal women. This may result from endogenous overproduction or over-replacement of thyroxine in women with hypothyroidism or those who receive thyroid-stimulating hormone (TSH)-suppressing thyroid hormone treatment for thyroid cancer. In contrast, the risk to bone seems to be minimal in women with primary hypothyroidism treated with thyroid hormone replacement without suppression of TSH. Women who present with hyperthyroidism should be screened for osteoporosis. Thyroxine replacement should be adjusted so that TSH is not suppressed. Thyroid replacement is not a contraindication for HRT but the dose of thyroxine may need to be increased because estrogen can increase concentrations of thyroxine-binding globulin. Conversely, the dose of thyroid replacement may need to be reduced when HRT is stopped.

Gastrointestinal disease

GALLBLADDER DISEASE

Gallbladder disease is a frequent problem in developed countries and is more common in women. Prevalence in large population surveys ranges from 5.9% to 21.9%. Gallbladder disease increases with age and obesity and the disease may be silent.

Two randomised trials (HERS and WHI) have shown an increased risk of gallbladder disease with oral HRT. The non-oral route is usually recommended in women with pre-existing disease but little evidence supports this.

LIVER DISEASE

Some types of liver disease, such as primary biliary cirrhosis, are associated with osteoporosis. A non-oral route of estrogen treatment is advised in women with liver disease to avoid the first liver pass but the evidence is limited.

CROHN'S DISEASE

Bone loss and osteoporosis are commonly reported in inflammatory bowel disease, especially Crohn's disease. Disease activity and corticosteriod therapy may be involved in the bone loss. Transdermal rather than oral HRT usually is preferred to ensure adequate absorption.

COELIAC DISEASE

Coeliac disease is also associated with an increased risk of fracture especially that of the hip. The mechanism that underlies osteoporosis in women with coeliac disease is likely to be related to calcium malabsorption, which leads to increased parathyroid hormone secretion, which, in turn, increases bone turnover and cortical bone loss. Malabsorption of vitamin D is probably of less importance. Again, transdermal rather than oral HRT is preferred.

Neurological disease

MIGRAINE

Migraine is predominantly a female disorder and is usually a condition of the reproductive years, starting during the teens and 20s. The lifetime prevalence of migraine may be as high as 25% in women compared with only 8% in men. It is unusual for migraines to start after the menopause. Menstruation often is a significant trigger and the perimenopause marks a time of increased migraine, usually with a decline in the postmenopause. HRT can help by stabilising fluctuations in estrogen that are associated with migraine. No good evidence supports the idea that HRT aggravates migraine. As migraine can be triggered by fluctuating concentrations of estrogen, the transdermal route is favoured over the oral route, because it produces more stable levels of estrogen. Unlike the contraceptive pill, no data suggest that the risk of ischaemic stroke is increased in women with migraine with aura who take HRT. Sequential progestogen treatment may be a trigger for migraine. The strategies that can be used are changing the type of progestogen (19-nortestosterone to 17-hydroxyprogesterone derivatives), changing to continuous combined therapy and delivering the progestogen transdermally or into the uterus with the levonorgestrel device. HRT can be given with treatments for migraine such as triptans.

EPILEPSY

Epilepsy is a common neurological disorder. In the laboratory, estrogen lowers and progesterone raises seizure threshold. Data about the menopause, HRT and epilepsy are limited. The number of women is small and the type and dose of HRT have not been examined systematically. No data as yet confirm whether the transdermal route is preferable to the oral route. Whether women who take oral therapy should take an increased dose (extrapolating from combined oral contraceptive usage) is not yet known. Of concern, anticonvulsant treatments can cause changes in calcium and bone metabolism leading to decreased bone mass with an increased risk of osteoporotic fractures. Phenytoin, carbamazepine and sodium valproate are recognised to affect metabolism of vitamin D and to have direct effects on bone cells that lead to impaired bone mass. Furthermore, some antiepileptics are inducers of liver enzymes and herbal preparations used for menopausal symptoms may interact with them.

PARKINSON'S DISEASE

The most prevalent serious movement disorder is Parkinson's disease, affecting about 1% of people over the age of 60 years. Men are more often affected than women. There is some evidence that estrogen may modify Parkinson manifestations. Women with Parkinson's disease sometimes report increased symptoms preceding or during menstruation, a time when circulating estrogen levels are at their lowest level. The observational literature on Parkinson's disease risk remains confusing with regard to menopause and HRT. The evidence regarding acute effects of HRT and Parkinson's disease is limited. Transdermal delivery of 17β-estradiol seems to display a slight prodopaminergic (that is, antiparkinsonian effect) without consistently altering dyskinesias. It would seem, therefore, that the use of HRT is not contraindicated.

DEPRESSION

Major and minor depressions are the two most prevalent forms of acute depressive illness. Major depression has an estimated lifetime prevalence of 17% and affects approximately twice as many women as men. The exact prevalence of minor depression is unclear, owing to differences in the diagnostic criteria; however, its prevalence is thought to approximate that of major depression. Perimenopausal depression is defined by the onset of depression at midlife in association with the onset of menstrual cycle irregularity or amenorrhoea. Epidemiological studies have found that the majority of postmenopausal women do not experience a major depression. Nevertheless, several community-based and clinic-based surveys suggest that the perimenopause is relevant to the development of affective disorders. Psychological problems reported during the menopause are likely to be related to previous problems. HRT is not contraindicated in women taking antidepressants.

Other conditions

ASTHMA

In women who have used systemic steroids, BMD needs to be assessed. There seems to be a small increase in the risk of asthma and asthma-like symptoms in women who use HRT. The use of HRT, however, does not seem to worsen pre-existing asthma. No evidence exists with regard to tibolone or raloxifene.

RENAL DISEASE

Patients with end-stage renal disease are at increased risk for early menopause, osteoporosis, cognitive dysfunction and cardiovascular disease. Interventions for preventing bone disease require further study.

AFTER TRANSPLANTATION

Transplantation is an established therapy for end-stage diseases of the kidney, endocrine pancreas, heart, liver and lung, and for many haematological disorders. Improved survival rates have been accompanied by increased recognition of previously neglected long-term complications of transplantation such as osteoporosis. The prevalence of osteopenia or osteoporosis may be as high as 80%. Pretransplantation bone disease and immunosuppressive therapy result in rapid bone loss and increased fracture rates early after transplantation. Post-transplant glucocorticoid therapy is thought to play a major role in reduction in bone mass. The additional role of other immunosuppressant treatments in bone loss is less clear but some evidence suggests that cyclosporin A and tacrolimus (FK506) produce osteopenia as a result of high bone turnover. Antiosteoporotic strategies such as bisphosphonates and vitamin D need to be considered but the data are limited.

OTOSCLEROSIS

This condition is inherited as a Mendelian dominant characteristic and leads to progressive deafness. Pregnancy can aggravate this condition and, rarely, it can worsen with oral contraceptives. No data, however, show that HRT causes a deterioration of the disease. As the natural course of the disease is progressive, it is likely that hearing will become more impaired in women who take HRT for many years.

MALIGNANT MELANOMA

This is a controversial area. It generally is accepted that no association exists between the risk of melanoma and the use of HRT. Reports about a relation between the prognosis of melanoma and HRT are contradictory. Estrogen receptors are present on melanomas, but it seems unlikely that estradiol has a direct effect on melanogenesis.

Lentigo maligna is the precursor of lentigo maligna melanoma. It is most common in the eighth decade, is found on the cheek or neck and correlates closely with exposure to ultraviolet radiation. That lentigo maligna possesses both estrogen and progesterone receptors suggests a possible role of these steroids in malignant transformation.

Further reading

CARDIOVASCULAR DISEASE AND VENOUS THROMBOEMBOLISM

Barrett-Connor E, Mosca L, Collins P, Geiger MJ, Grady D, Kornitzer M, et al; Raloxifene Use for The Heart (RUTH) Trial Investigators. Effects of raloxifene on cardiovascular events and breast cancer in postmenopausal women. N Engl J Med 2006;355:125–37.

British Heart Foundation [www.heartstats.org].

Canonico M, Oger E, Plu-Bureau G, Conard J, Meyer G, Lévesque H, et al; Estrogen and Thromboembolism Risk (ESTHER) Study Group. Hormone therapy and venous thromboembolism among postmenopausal women: impact of the route of estrogen administration and progestogens: the ESTHER study. Circulation 2007;115:840–5.

Cherry N, Gilmour K, Hannaford P, Heagerty A, Khan MA, Kitchener H, et al; ESPRIT team. Oestrogen therapy for prevention of reinfarction in postmenopausal women: a randomised placebo controlled trial. Lancet 2002;360:2001–8.

Clarke SC, Kelleher J, Lloyd-Jones H, Slack M, Schofield PM. A study of hormone replacement therapy in postmenopausal women with ischaemic heart disease: the Papworth HRT atherosclerosis study. BJOG 2002;109:1056–62.

Cummings SR. LIFT study is discontinued. BMJ 2006;332:667.

Curb JD, Prentice RL, Bray PF, Langer RD, Van Horn L, Barnabei VM, et al. Venous thrombosis and conjugated equine estrogen in women without a uterus. Arch Intern Med 2006;166:772–80.

Cushman M, Kuller LH, Prentice R, Rodabough RJ, Psaty BM, Stafford RS, et al; Women's Health Initiative Investigators. Estrogen plus progestin and risk of venous thrombosis. JAMA 2004;292:1573–80.

Grady D, Herrington D, Bittner V, Blumenthal R, Davidson M, Hlatky M, et al; HERS Research Group. Cardiovascular disease outcomes during 6.8 years of hormone therapy: Heart and Estrogen/progestin Replacement Study follow-up (HERS II). JAMA 2002;288(1):49–57.

Heron MP, Smith BL. Deaths: Leading causes for 2003. National Vital Statistics Report, Centers for Disease Control and Prevention [www.cdc.gov/nchs/products/pubs/pubd/hestats/leadingdeaths03/leadingdeaths03.htm].

Høibraaten E, Qvigstad E, Arnesen H, Larsen S, Wickstrøm E, Sandset PM. Increased risk of recurrent venous thromboembolism during hormone replacement therapy-results of the randomized, double-blind, placebo-controlled estrogen in venous thromboembolism trial (EVTET). *Thromb Haemost* 2000;84:961–7.

Royal College of Obstetricians and Gynaecologists. *Hormone Replacement Therapy and Venous Thromboembolism.* Green-top Guideline No. 19. London: RCOG; January 2004.

Hulley S, Grady D, Bush T, Furberg C, Herrington D, Riggs B, *et al.* Randomized trial of estrogen plus progestin for secondary prevention of coronary heart disease in postmenopausal women. Heart and Estrogen/progestin Replacement Study research group. *JAMA* 1998;280:605–13.

Lloyd GW. Heart disease and stroke. In: Rees M, Keith LG, editors. *Women Over 70: Where Normative Values do not Apply.* London: Informa Healthcare; 2007. p. 45–59.

Lobo RA. Surgical menopause and cardiovascular risks. *Menopause* 2007;14 (3 Suppl):562–6.

Løkkegaard E, Jovanovic Z, Heitmann BL, Keiding N, Ottesen B, Pedersen AT. The association between early menopause and risk of ischaemic heart disease: influence of hormone therapy. *Maturitas* 2006;53:226–33.

Schenck-Gustafsson K. Diagnosis of cardiovascular disease in women. *Menopause Int* 2007;13:19–22.

Rossouw JE, Anderson GL, Prentice RL. Risks and benefits of estrogen plus progestin in healthy postmenopausal women: principal results From the Women's Health Initiative randomized controlled trial. *JAMA* 2002;288:321–33.

Steiner AZ, Hodis HN, Lobo RA, Shoupe D, Xiang M, Mack WJ. Postmenopausal oral estrogen therapy and blood pressure in normotensive and hypertensive subjects: the Estrogen in the Prevention of Atherosclerosis Trial. *Menopause* 2005;12:728–33.

Swegle JM, Kelly MW. Tibolone: a unique version of hormone replacement therapy. *Ann Pharmacother* 2004;38:874–81.

Vasilakis C, Jick H, del Mar Melero-Montes M. Risk of idiopathic venous thromboembolism in users of progestagens alone. *Lancet* 1999;354:1610–11.

Viscoli CM, Brass LM, Kernan WN, Sarrel PM, Suissa S, Horwitz RI. A clinical trial of estrogen-replacement therapy after ischemic stroke. *N Engl J Med* 2001;345:1243–9.

Women's Health Initiative Steering Committee. Effects of conjugated equine estrogen in postmenopausal women with hysterectomy: the Women's Health Initiative randomized controlled trial. *JAMA* 2004;291:1701–12.

ENDOCRINE

Adeghate E, Schattner P, Dunn E. An update on the etiology and epidemiology of diabetes mellitus. *Ann N Y Acad Sci* 2006;1084:1–29.

Anderson KE, Anderson E, Mink PJ, Hong CP, Kushi LH, Sellers TA, *et al.* Diabetes and endometrial cancer in the Iowa women's health study. *Cancer Epidemiol Biomarkers Prev* 2001;10:611–16.

Arafah BM. Increased need for thyroxine in women with hypothyroidism during estrogen therapy. *N Engl J Med* 2001;344:1743–9.

Cummings SR, Nevitt MC, Browner WS, Stone K, Fox KM, Ensrud KE, *et al.* Risk factors for hip fracture in white women. Study of Osteoporotic Fractures Research Group. *N Engl J Med* 1995;332:767–73.

Eaton SE, Webster J, Allahabadia A. Thyroid disease and the menopausal woman. *J Br Menopause Soc* 2003;9:82–4.

Ferrara A, Quesenberry CP, Karter AJ, Njoroge CW, Jacobson AS, Selby JV; Northern California Kaiser Permanente Diabetes Registry. Current use of unopposed estrogen and estrogen plus progestin and the risk of acute myocardial infarction among women with diabetes: the Northern California Kaiser Permanente Diabetes Registry, 1995–1998. *Circulation* 2003;107:43–8.

Kanaya AM, Herrington D, Vittinghoff E, Lin F, Grady D, Bittner V, *et al.* Glycaemic effects of postmenopausal hormone therapy: the Heart and Estrogen/progestin Replacement Study. *Ann Intern Med* 2003;138:1–9.

Khoo CL, Perera M. Diabetes and the menopause. *J Br Menopause Soc* 2005;11:6–11.

Margolis KL, Bonds DE, Rodabough RJ, Tinker L, Phillips LS, Allen C, *et al.* Effect of oestrogen plus progestin on the incidence of diabetes in postmenopausal women: results from the Women's Health Initiative Hormone Trial. *Diabetologia* 2004;47:1175–87.

Nicodemus KK, Folsom AR. Type 1 and type 2 diabetes and incident hip fractures in postmenopausal women. *Diabetes Care* 2001;24:1192–7.

Pearce EN. Thyroid dysfunction in perimenopausal and postmenopausal women. *Menopause Int* 2007;13:8–13.

Rossi R, Origliani G, Modena M. Transdermal 17_ estradiol and risk of developing type 2 diabetes in a population of healthy, non obese postmenopausal women. *Diabetes Care* 2004;27:645–9.

Zendehdel K, Nyrén O, Ostenson CG, Adami HO, Ekbom A, Ye W. Cancer incidence in patients with type 1 diabetes mellitus: a population-based cohort study in Sweden. *J Natl Cancer Inst* 2003;95:1797–800.

GASTROINTESTINAL DISEASE

Cirillo DJ, Wallace RB, Rodabough RJ, Greenland P, LaCroix AZ, Limacher MC, *et al.* Effect of estrogen therapy on gallbladder disease. *JAMA* 2005;293:330–9.

Demerjian-Somogyi N, Palazzo E, Cohen-Solal M. Osteoporosis in patients with inflammatory bowel disease. *Joint Bone Spine* 2005;72:354–6.

Hay JE, Guichelaar MM. Evaluation and management of osteoporosis in liver disease. *Clin Liver Dis* 2005;9:747–66.

Hulley S, Grady D, Bush T, Furberg C, Herrington D, Riggs B, *et al.* Randomized trial of estrogen plus progestin for secondary prevention of coronary heart disease in postmenopausal women. Heart and Estrogen/progestin Replacement Study (HERS) Research Group. *JAMA* 1998;280:605–13.

Jahnsen J, Falch JA, Mowinckel P, Aadland E. Bone mineral density in patients with inflammatory bowel disease: a population-based prospective two-year follow-up study. *Scand J Gastroenterol* 2004;39:145–53.

Ludvigsson JF, Michaelsson K, Ekbom A, Montgomery SM. Coeliac disease and the risk of fractures – a general population-based cohort study. *Aliment Pharmacol Ther* 2007;25:273–85.

Shaffer EA. Gallstone disease: epidemiology of gallbladder stone disease. *Best Pract Res Clin Gastroenterol* 2006;20:981–96.

NEUROLOGICAL DISEASE

Bousser MG, Conard J, Kittner S, de Lignières B, MacGregor EA, Massiou H, *et al.* Recommendations on the risk of ischaemic stroke associated with use of combined oral contraceptives and hormone replacement therapy in women with migraine. International Headache Society Task Force on Combined Oral Contraceptives & Hormone Replacement Therapy. *Cephalalgia* 2000;20:155–6.

Currie LJ, Harrison MB, Trugman JM, Bennett JP, Wooten GF. Postmenopausal estrogen use affects risk for Parkinson disease. *Arch Neurol* 2004;61:886–8.

Henderson VW. The neurology of menopause. *Neurologist* 2006;12:149–59.

Dennerstein L, Guthrie JR, Clark M, Lehert P, Henderson VW. A population-based study of depressed mood in middle-aged, Australian-born women. *Menopause* 2004;11:563–8.

Freeman EW, Sammel MD, Liu L, Gracia CR, Nelson DB, Hollander L. Hormones and menopausal status as predictors of depression in women in transition to menopause. *Arch Gen Psychiatry* 2004;61:62–70.

Harden CL, Herzog AG, Nikolov BG, Koppel BS, Christos PJ, Fowler K, *et al.* Hormone replacement therapy in women with epilepsy: a randomized, double-blind, placebo-controlled study. *Epilepsia* 2006;47(9):1447–51.

MacGregor EA. Menstrual migraine. In: Rees M, Hope S, Ravnikar V, editors. *The Abnormal Menstrual Cycle.* Abingdon: Taylor and Francis; 2005. p. 197–218.

Schmidt PJ, Rubinow DR. Reproductive ageing, sex steroids and depression. *J Br Menopause Soc* 2006;12(4):178–85.

OTHER

Barr RG, Wentowski CC, Grodstein F, Somers SC, Stampfer MJ, Schwartz J, *et al.* Prospective study of postmenopausal hormone use and newly diagnosed asthma and chronic obstructive pulmonary disease. *Arch Intern Med* 2004;164:379–86.

Ebeling PR. Transplantation osteoporosis. *Curr Osteoporos Rep* 2007;5:29–37.

Naldi L, Altieri A, Imberti GL, Giordano L, Gallus S, La Vecchia C; Oncology Study Group of the Italian Group for Epidemiologic Research in Dermatology (GISED). Cutaneous malignant melanoma in women. Phenotypic characteristics, sun exposure, and hormonal factors: a case–control study from Italy. *Ann Epidemiol* 2005;15:545–50.

Palmer SC, Strippoli GF, McGregor DO. Interventions for preventing bone disease in kidney transplant recipients: a systematic review of randomized controlled trials. *Am J Kidney Dis* 2005;45:638–49.

Persson I, Yuen J, Bergkvist L, Schairer C. Cancer incidence and mortality in women receiving estrogen and estrogen-progestin replacement therapy: long-term follow-up of a Swedish cohort. *Int J Cancer* 1996;67:327–32.

Thompson W. Otosclerosis and hormone replacement therapy: fact or fiction? *J Br Menopause Soc* 1999;5:54.

Troisi RJ, Speizer FE, Willett WC, Trichopoulos D, Rosner B. Menopause, postmenopausal estrogen preparations, and the risk of adult-onset asthma. A prospective cohort study. *Am J Respir Crit Care Med* 1995;152:1183–8.

Index